TIGER WOODS'S BACK AND TOMMY JOHN'S ELBOW

INJURIES AND TRAGEDIES THAT TRANSFORMED CAREERS, SPORTS, AND SOCIETY

JONATHAN GELBER, MD, MS

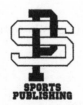

SPORTS
PUBLISHING

Sports Publishing books may be purchased in bulk at special discounts for sales promotion, corporate gifts, fund-raising, or educational purposes. Special editions can also be created to specifications. For details, contact the Special Sales Department, Sports Publishing, 307 West 36th Street, 11th Floor, New York, NY 10018 or sportspubbooks@skyhorsepublishing.com.

Sports Publishing® is a registered trademark of Skyhorse Publishing, Inc.®, a Delaware corporation.

Visit our website at www.sportspubbooks.com.

10 9 8 7 6 5 4 3 2 1

Library of Congress Cataloging-in-Publication Data is available on file.

Cover design by Tom Lau
Cover photo credit Associated Press (Tiger Woods) and Getty Images

ISBN: 978-1-68358-258-8
Ebook ISBN: 978-1-68358-259-5

Printed in the United States of America

To my four amazing and unique children,
Liam, Odin, Noah, and Ella

Contents

Introduction **The Cobra Effect**　vii

1) **Sandy Koufax, Tommy John, and an Epidemic**　1

2) **The Magic and Cookie Johnson Effect**　15

3) **Lyle Alzado and the Steroid Conversation**　43

4) **Len Bias and "Biased" Drug Laws**　63

5) **Hank Gathers, Dale Lloyd, and Athlete Screening**　79

6) **Ayrton Senna, Dale Earnhardt, and NASCAR's Car of Tomorrow**　95

7) **Duk-koo Kim and Boxing's Biggest Tragedy**　115

8) **Tom Brady and Protecting the Quarterback**　137

9) **Tiger's Back**　157

References and Sources Used　177

INTRODUCTION
The Cobra Effect

LEGEND HAS IT THAT DURING the time of colonial India, when the land was ruled by the British crown, a concern grew among the local leaders of Delhi. They approached the British Raj with whispers of a slow venomous snake invasion. Among the invaders was one snake that was the most feared of all—the mighty cobra. Even today, few animals ignite such a level of fear simply by raising their heads. Dabs of color speckle across its broad head and harken back to the crowns of pharaohs. A simple flick of its forked tongue warns all who approach of its dagger-like fatal quickness. For centuries, the only weapon in India against these fearsome creatures was the droning sound of snake charmers. Wrapped in turbans and surrounded by baskets, these mysterious men seemed to hypnotize the formidable creature's gaze aided only by a musical instrument. Despite their temporary powers of control, these men did nothing to defeat the snake and its invasion. They neither hunted nor killed them. As traditional mystic healers, many of them were trained to handle snakes, and snake bites, but their skill set levied no control over the snake population. And so the number of snakes grew, as did the local leaders' concern.

The British Raj had an idea. Like any dangerous outlaw demanded, a bounty would be placed on the cobra snake. The people of Delhi would turn against the invading force. They would be rewarded for bringing the Raj the skins of dead cobras. Surely, thought the local leaders, this would solve the problem of too many poisonous snakes. It began with a trickle, but soon a deluge of rewards was being handed out as baskets with snake skins piled up.

At first, the Raj and local leaders were proud of what unfolded. Clearly, they were winning the war. The cobra population was withering by the basketload. And yet whispers fluttered in the background. The bounty didn't seem to be making much difference. The snakes still tormented the villages. Were there really that many snakes to be caught in the first place? How big was this cobra invasion really?

Then the whispers grew into rumors and reached the Raj himself. Where were these snakes coming from? Were they really wild? So the Raj sent local leaders out into the villages to investigate. It didn't take long for the local government to uncover the plot. The people of Delhi were breeding cobras on their own in order to kill them and turn the snakeskins in for the reward money. Once the Raj learned of this subterfuge, he immediately scrapped the reward program. As the news of the reward program's cancellation spread from village to village, the snake breeders became very angry. What were they to do now with thousands of unwanted and unvaluable cobras? Without a market to sell them, they released the black reptiles. The freed snakes slithered into the wild and spread across the villages. With that, the wild cobra population in Delhi skyrocketed, resulting in the exact opposite consequence than the original program had intended. In the end, the reactive solution crafted by the Raj actually ended up making the problem worse.

This story has since been used to illustrate what happens when an attempted solution to a problem results in an unintended consequence. As with the case of the Raj's reward program, the consequence can even make the original problem worse. When this happens, it is dubbed "The Cobra Effect." We often recognize that sometimes things just don't go how we expected. We can plan for all contingencies and have the best intentions in mind, but sometimes these best-laid plans can result in unintended consequences. We miss connections to other parties. We fail to plan for the long term. We may simply swap out one problem for another. We can even misinterpret the data in front of us. And other times, we may miss an opportunity to address a problem before it becomes bigger. These mistakes are all part of being human. But oftentimes it makes sense to take a step back and focus on the big picture; then maybe, armed with the knowledge that unintended consequences do exist, we can start to win our own battle against the cobra. This book explores various examples of the Cobra Effect in the world of sports and what lessons we can glean and apply going forward.

1
Sandy Koufax, Tommy John, and an Epidemic

ASK ANY DOCTOR OR JOURNALIST to name an injury that changed the face of sports as we know it, and invariably the name Tommy John comes to mind. Tommy John surgery, or "TJ" surgery as some call it, has become the subject of numerous books and countless articles as more and more professional pitchers undergo what is considered a "career-saving" surgery. Yet, the story does not stop there. In fact, despite, or possibly because of, the career-saving surgery, we are amidst an epidemic. So much so, that both the major league pitcher Tommy John and his own son are worried about today's teenagers. The term the 288-win pitcher uses is "appalling." But to fully understand the story of the surgery that was first performed on the elder Tommy John in 1974, we have to go back a decade earlier.

On April 22, 1964, the defending national champion Los Angeles Dodgers were in the midst of a six-game losing streak when they faced off midweek against the St. Louis Cardinals. That Wednesday, Sandy Koufax, the National League's most valuable player, struggled almost immediately. It was only one inning in, but a crowd of 31,410, one of the largest to see a home opener in St. Louis, was already on its feet. Koufax had struck out the first two Cardinals, but the third batter, Bill White, managed to get to first thanks to a wild third strike that sailed past the catcher. The next batter, Ken Boyer, was walked on four straight pitches. It was two outs with two men on, and the Cardinals' Charley James stepped to the plate. Koufax battled to a count of two balls and two strikes. He threw the next pitch high and away. The batter reached out, swung, and connected, sending the ball to the opposite-field rooftop. The crowd roared as Koufax gave up a three-run homer.

When the inning was finally over, the left-hander returned to the dugout and began to complain about his throwing elbow. It was a culmination of weeks of pain he had been trying to grit his teeth and play through. Later in the dressing room, Koufax, with an icepack on his injured arm, would tell the Associated Press, "It hurts like heck. I've had it for three weeks. I haven't had anything on the ball in any of my starts. I was just lucky to get by until now. But it got me out there tonight."

The Cardinals' team physician I.C. Middleman had taken a look at the Dodger's arm at the end of the game. "He [Koufax] was visibly hurt when he threw that wild third strike," the Cardinals' team physician remarked to the AP. He diagnosed Koufax's injuries as "medial epicondylitis" (inflammation of the inner side of the elbow) coupled with a slight forearm muscle tear. Despite describing Koufax's arm as "rigid and just like a hot dog," he reassured everyone that it wasn't too serious. Fresh off the Dodgers losing their seventh straight game, Koufax was sent packing back home to Los Angeles, where he could be evaluated by the Dodgers' team physician, Robert Kerlan.

Based on what we know today about pitchers and elbow injuries, it's likely that Koufax suffered the same injury that would sideline Tommy John one decade later. If you look at the elbow simply as two bones connected, with one bone above (the humerus) and one bone below (the ulna), the joint they make looks like a hinge. It opens and closes in a smooth fashion (we won't talk about rotation and the other forearm bone here); but when a pitcher winds back to throw the ball, he has to bring his arm back as far as possible, like a medieval catapult. He has to generate enough power and momentum to launch the ball forward.

In this position, when the elbow is cocked back, it is no longer acting as a hinge. In this case, it's actually bending sideways, and that places significant stress along the inner (medial) side of the elbow. If you look at still photographs of professional pitchers, it looks like their elbows bend sideways almost 90 degrees. To keep the joint from opening up that way, the body has a small ligament that connects the two bones called the ulnar collateral ligament, or UCL for short. Amazingly, despite its small size, this ligament is able to withstand pretty sizeable forces.

Now, before proceeding any further, we should take a quick pause to point out the difference between tendons and ligaments. A ligament is a thick, rope-like structure that runs from one bone to another and helps to stabilize a joint. We will talk about the ACL, which is a ligament connecting the knee bones, in another chapter. In contrast, a tendon is not a freestanding structure. It's actually the part of a muscle that attaches to the bone. A muscle starts out as big, red, and meaty, but before it connects to a bone, it transitions into a small white tendon. This way, when the muscle part contracts, it pulls the tendon part, and since the tendon is attached to the bone, the bone moves. That's how we make our joints bend and rotate.

Baseball pitching is a complex task that starts at the ground and works its way up through multiple joints. When you pitch, you really should use your whole body, something scientists term the "kinetic chain." It requires training the human body to be an amazingly efficient machine. To become an effective pitcher, an athlete must be able to generate high levels of arm speed. The average shoulder rotation for a high-level pitcher is anywhere from about 6,200 to 7,200 degrees/sec. Since 360 degrees equals one circle, that's the equivalent of the shoulder going all the way around almost twenty times in one second. With the arm back and the elbow bent like a hinge at 90 degrees, the small band of tissue from the UCL is responsible for 55 percent of the resistance to stretching across the inner side of the elbow. What's even scarier is that during a pitch, the forces across the elbow actually meet or exceed the mechanical strength of just ligament itself. With every throw, the ligament teeters on the brink of destruction and therefore relies on the muscles, bones, and perhaps most important, proper pitching technique to protect it.

So now that we know what's happening at the elbow joint in a pitcher, let's turn our attention back to Koufax's arm. Dr. Kerlan regularly treated Koufax's elbow pain for several years with ice baths, multiple cortisone injections, and anti-inflammatory pills. He even turned to using capsaicin cream derived from hot peppers meant to kill the nerves that sense pain. The cream was so potent that Carroll Beringer, Koufax's teammate, accidentally put on Koufax's shirt during a game in St. Louis and soon after was struck with skin blistering, nausea, and vomiting. Koufax's elbow pain became so severe that he turned to using Phenylbutazone, a potent anti-inflammatory. Phenylbutazone was originally approved for human use in 1949 but soon after its release was considered unsafe in humans due to its effect on white blood cells and bone marrow. Multiple deaths in the 1950s were linked to its use. It still found a home, however, as one of the most common anti-inflammatories used in horses.

As Koufax's elbow joint, and likely UCL, suffered years of repetitive injury without stabilization, the cartilage in Koufax's elbow would wear away, leading to life-altering arthritis. In a 1999 *Sports Illustrated* article, Tom Verducci described Koufax during his pitching years as unable to straighten his left arm. His elbow was curved like a parenthesis, and he had to have a tailor shorten the left sleeve on all his coats. Even daily tasks were difficult, as Verducci described: "On bad days he'd have to bend his neck to get his face closer to his left hand so that he could shave. And on the worst days he had to shave with his right hand. He still held his fork in his left hand, but sometimes he had to bend closer to the plate to get the food into his mouth." There's something about seeing legendary sports stars struggle with menial daily tasks that really drives home the sacrifice they made to their sport.

In 1966, at the early age of 30, Koufax decided to retire from baseball after what had already been a Hall of Fame career. Still, fans of Sandy Koufax wonder how many more records he would have set if his elbow didn't fall apart. Koufax's elbow attrition, however, gave Robert Kerlan a front-row seat to the degradation that can happen to a pitcher's elbow when it becomes destabilized from a torn ligament. So when he brought on his younger partner Frank Jobe into what eventually became known as the Kerlan-Jobe Clinic, it provided Jobe his own connection to Koufax and the LA Dodgers.

Kerlan would officially take the reins as head team physician in 1968, and, four years later, Tommy John left the Chicago White Sox to join the Dodgers. By the time Tommy arrived on the team, he was already no stranger to elbow injury and pain. Even as far back as age thirteen, when he transitioned from a Little League field to a full-size baseball field, his elbow would swell up from pitching. He would continue to pitch and rely on his elbow surviving for the next 18 years—until one fateful day on July 17, 1974.

On that day, Tommy John was already one year older than Koufax's age when he retired. He was on the mound against the Montreal Expos. The scoreboard signaled there was one out. With runners behind him on first and second base, he knew what he wanted to do. He would throw a sinker to force the batter to hit a ground ball. With the ball rolling on the ground, he could easily scoop it up and throw it to third, setting up a double play. They would turn an easy two outs and get out of the inning. Setting himself up to field the return hit, Tommy let the pitch fly. Out of nowhere, he felt a searing pain across the inside of his elbow. The ball barely made it across the plate. He tried to throw another pitch but had nothing on it. He signaled to the manager to take him out of the game.

He walked over to the dugout, went down to the bench, and grabbed his jacket. He turned to their trainer and told him something's wrong. They needed Dr. Jobe. Up until that point, the pitcher had amassed an impressive record of 13–3 for the season. Hoping they could get him back for the rest of the season, Jobe instructed him to rest his elbow for a month. After the prescribed time off, John tried to pitch again but found that his pain still hadn't subsided.

Tommy's elbow was unstable, and no matter how much he rested it, he couldn't do his job as a pitcher. Jobe thought long and hard about how he could reconstruct the important UCL ligament and restabilize the elbow. He did not want to resign Tommy to Koufax's fate. Instead, he wanted to surgically thread a tendon through the bones of the elbow where the UCL used to be. He talked with Dr. Herbert Stark, a hand surgeon he'd brought in for advice, who suggested he could use a muscle in the forearm called the palmaris longus. It has a long, narrow tendon that would be perfect for threading through bone tunnels. You can actually see your own palmaris tendon pop up in the middle of the palm-side of your wrist if you touch your thumb and pinky finger together (note: 16 percent of you won't have it in at least one hand).

Jobe went on to perform the landmark surgery on Tommy John that same year of 1974. John began to feel better but soon developed numbness in his ring and small fingers. About a month later, he underwent a more secretive second surgery to free up scar tissue around the ulnar nerve. This "funny-bone" nerve runs along the same side of the elbow as the UCL all the way down to the pinky and ring fingers. After the nerve was freed up, John returned to rehabbing his elbow. Known for his "sinkball" pitching, he would work with his teammate and fellow pitcher Mike Marshall, who himself had a PhD in kinesiology. Together, the two of them crafted a different way of pitching to protect his arm. John returned to the Dodgers in 1976, more than one year after the surgery, and continued to pitch until 1989, achieving over half of his career wins after the surgery. This year-long rehab has been shown to be very common after this surgery, and, like John and his teammate Marshall discovered, if surgery is one-half of injury recovery, focusing on pitching mechanics is the other half.

Besides saving Tommy John's career, though, the elbow reconstruction surgery also permeated the media and shed light on what was a devastating problem. It would bear the pitcher's own name and be nicknamed "Tommy John" surgery. But this is where we encounter the dark side of this story—the unexpected Cobra Effect. Unfortunately, in today's ever-competitive baseball era, the "career-saving" aspect of the surgery has been misunderstood and overplayed by media, coaches, players, and parents. In 2010, Yankees team physician and Columbia University orthopedic surgeon Chris Ahmad published the results of a survey of 189 high school and collegiate players, 15 coaches, and 31 parents via either one-on-one interviews or a mail-in questionnaire. His research team asked them their thoughts and feelings about Tommy John surgery. What they found was alarming. Half of the high school athletes wrongly believed that the elbow surgery should be performed in the absence of injury with the sole intention to improve performance. Despite numerous studies showing increased risk of injury based on the total number of pitches thrown in a game and accumulated over the course of a year, 31 percent of coaches wrongly believed that the number of pitches thrown was not a risk factor for injury to the elbow ligament. And many more underestimated the time it took to recover from surgery by several months.

A similar study was published in 2015 in an effort to learn what members of the MLB media understood about elbow injuries. The authors of the study used Survey Monkey to email a survey to over 1,000 members of the media including print, Internet, radio, and/or television who were directly involved in the coverage of Major League Baseball. Five hundred sixteen people completed the anonymous online survey, which represented about 47 percent of the emails sent out. Below are some of the questions from the actual survey that you can ask yourself:

1) How often are professional pitchers able to return to play professional baseball after Tommy John Surgery? (Pick a percentage)

2) Does Tommy John surgery improve PITCHING CONTROL compared to other pitchers without surgery?
__Yes __No __I Don't Know

3) Does Tommy John surgery DECREASE PAIN with throwing?
__Yes __No __I Don't Know

4) In general, Tommy John surgery should be performed for (check all that apply):
___Shoulder Ligament ___Shoulder ___Elbow Ligament
___Elbow
___Decreased Throwing Velocity and Poor Control

5) Does an athlete need to have an elbow injury to have Tommy John surgery?
___Yes ___No ___I Don't Know

6) Are throwing injuries preventable?
___Yes ___No ___I Don't Know

7) Throwing injuries are related to: (select all that apply)
___Number of Pitches ___Type of Pitch ___Velocity ___Accuracy
___Overuse

8) Are pitch counts important for prevention of Tommy John surgery?
___Yes ___No ___I Don't Know

Source: Conte SA, Hodgins JL, ElAttrache NS, Patterson-Flynn N, Ahmad CS. "Media Perceptions of Tommy John Surgery." *Phys Sportsmed*. 2015 Nov; 43(4):375–80.

What the authors found was rather sobering. Almost half (45 percent) of those who responded to the survey did not know if an athlete needed an elbow injury as a prerequisite for UCL reconstruction. That's about the same proportion of high school athletes who responded to the 2012 study. Furthermore, 25 percent of the media polled believed the primary indication for the surgery was performance enhancement—which is absolutely false. Furthermore, only slightly less than half of those members of the media surveyed believed the use of pitch counts to be important in the prevention of UCL injury, and one-third felt that throwing injuries were not preventable in adolescent baseball.

The issue of pitch counts is not something to be ignored or misunderstood. Pitch counts based on age, number of innings, and days of rest were something world-renowned orthopedic surgeon and elbow surgery expert James Andrews and his Birmingham, Alabama, team established and promoted after seeing firsthand the Tommy John surgery epidemic in teenagers. It was Andrews who was one of the first surgeons to speak out about the alarming number of teenagers he saw in his operating room undergoing UCL reconstruction. His team's research showed one of the greatest risk factors for injuring your elbow as a youth pitcher was related to the number of pitches you threw in a game.

In late August 2006, Little League became the first national youth baseball organization to institute a pitch count. The Little League International Board of Directors approved the measure unanimously at its annual meeting two days before the Little League Baseball World Series concluded. For the two years prior to the ruling, Little League conducted a Pitch Count Pilot Program to determine the feasibility of implementing a regulation limiting the number of pitches a Little Leaguer could throw in a day as well as the required rest before pitching again. Fifty leagues were studied in 2005, and nearly 500 programs were involved in 2006.

Surveys of those leagues showed the overwhelming majority were able to implement a pitch count without any problems. They found that they were able to develop other pitchers who might not have otherwise ever taken the mound. They also found that their pitchers were stronger at the end of the season, with less arm pain. Previously, Little League pitching regulations limited pitchers in age 12 and under leagues to six innings per week (Sunday through Saturday) and six innings per game but did not focus on the number of total pitches thrown. The number of innings allowed was increased for older age groups, but again the total number of pitches was not taken into consideration.

Nevertheless, at the upper levels above Little League, there has been a resistance to implementing pitch counts. Some opponents feel that pitch counts favor larger schools or larger rosters with deeper benches over smaller schools. Coaches at larger schools have more reserve pitchers, while coaches with smaller rosters may not have the number of pitchers needed to make it through a season. Sometimes coaches and managers are too focused on winning to recognize when a player needs to be taken out of the rotation to rest or heal for a few days. Similarly, the most talented athletes are usually very competitive by nature and are reluctant to tell their coaches when they need to come out of the game. They may make the grievous mistake of continuing to throw even when their elbow hurts. They are more focused on how many strikeouts or "Ks" they can achieve than how many pitches they throw. They also don't want to let their team down. And these pitch counts don't even come into play during warm-ups, bullpen, and practice.

Other risk factors for injury the Birmingham group and other researchers have found include: pitching for more than one team at a time, playing baseball year-round without a three-month break in a row from baseball itself (playing other sports has been deemed okay), and pitching at showcases. Showcases have been traditionally used as a way for an athlete to show his or her talents to scouts, but they often occur during the off-season. As a result, the pitchers are either not physically prepared to give a full effort, or, if they are pitching year-round, they lack the adequate time to recover between seasons.

John Manuel was an editor-in-chief of *Baseball America*, a magazine that covers baseball at every level, with a particular focus on up-and-coming players. He is also a scout for the professional Minnesota Twins club and understands that showcases do provide scouts an opportunity for better players to face better pitchers more often than they would in plain old high school baseball, but he feels we need to work on better regulation of when and how often they occur. Manuel puts some of the onus on the organizers and scouts: "I think showcases are needed, but there are just too many of them, and at all times of year. Scouts could make an impact by not going to showcases that are held during difficult times of year." However, he puts the final emphasis on education. "But at some point," he says. "It's up to the players and parents to inform themselves."

Regarding Tommy John surgery improving performance, the statistics are not much in support of the mythical enhancement. In 2007, a group from the Penn Sports Medicine Center looked at 68 major league pitchers who pitched in at least one major league game before undergoing UCL reconstruction between 1998 and 2003. The authors then looked at statistics such as mean innings pitched and earned run average (ERA) before and after UCL surgery. They found that 82 percent of the pitchers returned to the majors after surgery, but it took about 18.5 months. Once they were back, there weren't any changes in their ERA. By the second season after surgery, these high-level pitchers were back to the same average innings pitched for the season. They were no better or worse by two years out from surgery. However, 8 percent of them never made it back.

A few years later, in 2014, the University of Chicago published a study looking at ball velocity following UCL reconstruction. They ended up identifying 38 MLB pitchers, eight of whom never made it back to pitching in the majors. Eventually, they whittled down the selection to 28 pitchers. The researchers then looked at data that had been collected by MLB since 2007 using a tool called PITCHf/x. This tool tracks almost all pitches thrown during each official game and records pitch velocity. They found that in the first year back, pitchers had lost a little over 1 mph off their fastball and changeup. By the second year back, they had begun to lose 1 mph in their curveball, which continued to decline into the third year back. The only pitch that didn't decline statistically was the slider. However, when the authors compared these declines to pitchers who did not have UCL reconstruction, their performance decrease was no different. So, while they lost some speed off their fastball, curveball, and changeup, so did the nonsurgery group. What they didn't do was increase their pitch speed.

A larger study in 2014 was done by Columbia University wherein they looked back at 147 MLB pitchers who had UCL reconstruction surgery. They found that 80 percent returned to pitch in at least one

MLB game, but only 67 percent managed to return to the same level and 57 percent actually ended up back on the disabled list because of their throwing arms. Again, most statistics such as ERA and fastball velocity declined compared to the season before surgery, but no different from other nonsurgical pitchers in the league.

Only one study really showed an improvement after UCL reconstruction surgery. This study was also performed in 2014, out of Rush Medical Center in Chicago. When they looked back at MLB pitchers, they were less restrictive in their inclusion criteria than the other studies. They also used different criteria to compare to pitchers who did not have surgery. As a result, they found that pitchers who had undergone UCL reconstruction actually showed improvements in some areas such as lower ERAs and allowing fewer home runs. It is important, though, to recognize that a lot of baseball statistics that focus on the pitcher are often dictated by how the fielders play behind them.

Since the demands of pitching might be more pronounced in analyzing the after-effects of UCL reconstruction surgery, researchers have also looked at position players. In a study out of Houston, Texas, all the MLB players who underwent UCL reconstructions between 1984 and 2015 from available records were recorded. Out of that number, 38 players who were active in the majors for at least a year before or after their surgery were identified. The percentage of players who returned to sports (RTS) by position is shown in the following table:

Position	Return to Sport Percentage	Average Days to Return to Sport
Catcher	71.4	280 +/- 100.2
Infielder	91.7	362 +/- 144.9
Outfielder	85.7	337.3 +/- 107.4
Overall	84.8	336.9 +/- 121.8

Data from: "Performance and Return to Sport after Tommy John Surgery among Major League Baseball Position Players." Jack RA et al. *AJSM* 46 (7) 2018.

Outfielders had the highest rate of UCL reconstruction of position players. They made up 14 out of the 33 players studied. Of those who did return, many had to change positions. Forty-eight percent had to adjust usually to a position that required less forceful throws over a shorter distance. The one position that didn't seem to change was catcher, but that also may be because it is a highly specialized role with little interchangeability within the team roster.

Unfortunately, in our society, many kids are being pushed too hard to the point of breaking down, and the media have not helped spread the word of injury prevention. Journalists in the field are trained in reporting stories, but not trained in medical info. And frankly, it's not necessarily on their to-do list. And when it comes to certain sports organizations, some on the inside will tell you it's easier to send an injured player to the world-famous elbow surgeon than it is to implement an organization- or team-wide injury prevention program.

So, while we can trace Koufax's injury to Dr. Robert Kerlan and Kerlan to Dr. Frank Jobe and helping heal Tommy John's elbow, we can also trace this elbow injury lineage one step further to misinformation and a current youth sports injury epidemic. That's where the cobra coils up and settles atop the pitcher's mound. The idea that we can "save" a pitcher's elbow, coupled with other misinformation, has given some in the sport a green light to pitch until their elbow gives out.

The group that is perhaps at greatest risk for injury in baseball is the youth. Whether it's to gain a meal ticket for the family, to meet unfulfilled dreams of the parents, or simply in the well-intentioned spirit of enjoyment, children are beginning to adopt a pattern of single-sport specialization earlier and earlier in their lives. It is estimated that more than 6 million adolescents participate in organized baseball in the United States. Sports medicine physicians are starting to see younger and younger patients in their clinics for overuse injuries, and doctors and trainers are currently seeing what amounts to an "epidemic" of younger patients undergoing elbow reconstruction surgery that was once relegated to professional pitchers. Of the Tommy John surgeries that were performed in the US from 2007 to 2011, 56.8 percent were performed on 15-to-19-year-olds, which was more than double the percentage that was performed on 20-to-24-year-olds. In New York

State alone, the number of Tommy John surgeries performed between 2003 and 2014 increased by 343 percent. And recent data suggest that the trend will continue. Famed surgeon James Andrews describes the increased Tommy John surgery problem this way: "When I started in this career I never imagined it would become routine for a fifteen-year-old to undergo such drastic treatment."

Jeff Passan is a baseball journalist for Yahoo! Sports and the author of the 2016 *New York Times* bestselling book *The Arm*, in which he follows two pitchers recovering from UCL surgery. The book's intention was to both educate the public, but also send up a warning signal to parents, players, and coaches. The bestselling author's experience could be described as sobering, not only during the research and writing of his book, but also afterward during its promotion. "I was most disappointed with the complicity and irresponsibility of adults," Passan said. "It's a combination of ignorance, vicarious living, and evils—I don't use these words lightly. It's parents who don't know any better and coaches who are unwilling or don't know how to teach them."

So if someone like Passan, a sports journalist with strong media connections, can write a bestselling book on the very topic of the elbow injury crises, why isn't the information getting to the intended audience? His hypothesis, based on his experience, is that the parents' effort to educate themselves may be lacking, or perhaps they are just ignorant of the risk factors. He recalls one very telling moment: "I was at Yankee Stadium for a trade show and a woman told me her son plays baseball at 9 and is a pitcher who struck out 11. So in our conversation, I calculated he probably threw 70 to 80 pitches and I told her about it. And she had no clue he could be getting hurt at that age."

So in the end, we have to ask ourselves, if Dr. Kerlan never took care of Sandy Koufax, and Dr. Jobe never saved Tommy John's career, would we be operating on and "saving the arm" of 15-year-old pitchers today? Like the cobra snakes of India, have we released more of the very problem we were combating back into the wild?

2

The Magic and
Cookie Johnson Effect

WHILE COBRAS MAY HAVE BEEN the problem in India, Indochina had a different animal foe on their hands. What is now called Vietnam was in the late 19th century referred to as French Indochina and was under the rule of a Governor-General. In 1897, France appointed Paul Doumer to the post in an attempt to modernize the capital, Hanoi. From 1897 to 1902, Doumer reshaped the infrastructure of the French colony. By the time he was done, the citizens of the city could walk along wide tree-lined avenues on their way to beautiful French colonial buildings for business before retiring to their new and spacious, multi-room homes. One of the longest bridges in Asia was erected, connecting the Hoan Kiem and Long Bien districts across the Red River. The Grand Palais de l'Exposition was built to house Hanoi's world exhibition fair that same year.

An especially momentous amenity was the installation of toilets in many of the new homes. These toilets were all connected to an intricate and vast sewer system that was designed underground. Yet, while the shiny new city sparkled aboveground, something was brewing in the dark underbelly of the sewers belowground. In the cool, damp, and isolated environment created by the pipes, sewer rats could breed and grow in relative safety. Soon, the rat colony multiplied exponentially and began to expand its borders. As the border zones crept farther and farther in all directions, it did not take long for them to overlap with the French section of town. Before long, the rodent invaders began to make their presence known. They appeared on the streets. They ran through the spacious villas. They were everywhere. The problem didn't stop with just the nuisance of their presence scurrying about. The rats brought with them fleas and *Yersinia pestis*, the bacterial agent of the Bubonic plague. As a consequence of the rat infestation, a public health crisis burgeoned.

Alarmed by the developments, the colonial administration called a meeting to address the problem. They needed to curtail the ever-multiplying rat problem. Their solution was to establish a new occupation, namely, that of local rat hunter. They would hire people from the villages of Hanoi and create their own army to combat the rats. The mission of the soldiers would be a simple one. They would descend into the dark and damp sewers and kill as many rats as they could. In the beginning, it was a simple but effective offensive. At one point during the onslaught, 10,000 to 20,000 rats were killed every single day the campaign took place. And yet, the vermin continued to multiply and invade.

At this point, a larger army was solicited, and any Vietnamese citizen with a penchant for rodent bloodshed could descend into the subterranean war zone. As proof of their destruction, the rat hunters would return with souvenirs of rat-tails, one for each rat that met its demise. The incoming stream of rat-tails for reward was steady and bountiful. It seemed like the French were winning the war, but soon it became apparent to any observer that the numbers of rats running amok did not decrease. In fact, not only was their population increasing, so was the sight of rats without tails. It turns out, it's easier to just chop off the tail of a rat than to actually trap and kill it. And by letting it live, it could breed more rats—rats with more valuable tails for the bounty. Just like the case back in India, the animals began to be farmed simply for the reward of turning in a tail. Left without another option, the campaign was called off. Soon, more cases of the bubonic plague appeared, cascading into to a full-blown outbreak. By this point in 1906, Paul Doumer was back home in France pursuing his political career. Twenty-five years later, he would be assassinated, one year into his term as President of France.

What the Hanoi Rat Problem has shown us is that you can get public buy-in and participation for the right cause, but if you are using the wrong marker for progress, you might be missing the actual picture. Your strategy might end up being misguided or fruitless. You might feel like you're getting immediate results, but if you aren't measuring the right thing, what you think is progress may actually just be a splash in the bucket. Therein, we find our next Cobra Effect.

EACH BOUNCE OF THE BASKETBALL echoed throughout the arena. Pregame setup was starting, but he was no longer the center of the frenzy. He could close his eyes and still see the flashbulbs going off in L.A.'s Great Western Forum every time he touched the ball. He felt like a king on the court. The crowd would scream his name at the top of their lungs. He could feel their collective breaths all around him, mixed with the perspiration of the game. The perspiration that he knew didn't carry any disease. Yet, no matter how much he or the doctors or the media or the team's own athletic trainer told the other players that HIV was not contagious through sweat, there were still whispers and double-takes. What he missed most, though, was the one-on-one. That feeling of the other player knocking him around and him giving it back; it was like two gladiators battling for supremacy. But nobody wanted to bang around with him anymore. Not since his announcement and retirement two months before.

It was about 5 p.m. on January 5, 1992, and Rony Seikaly was shooting around at the other end of the court, himself recovering from an injury. Seikaly, a standout player for the Miami Heat, had watched his own cousin die from blood-tranfusion-related AIDS in 1986. He knew what it was like for an HIV and AIDS patient to feel ostracized—to be treated as less than human. So the 6'11" center did what he knew how to do best. He walked over to the other side of the court and began shooting baskets. At first, he just shot around with the other player. Two players playing in parallel. Before long, though, he mustered up the courage to challenge the other player to a game of one-on-one. They played with all they had. And they played for real. Full-contact one-on-one basketball for 30 straight minutes, giving bumps and taking them. The gathering crowd and the media watched. The other players stopped what they were doing. All the eyes in the arena turned to him. And for a few moments, Magic Johnson felt at home again.

"Hoo hoo hoo," growled the studio audience, their fists pumping in the air. Magic stood in front of them in an oversize light-colored suit, clapping, pointing, and beaming his trademark smile. It was two months prior to that most important one-on-one game. He was walking out on the set of his close friend Arsenio Hall's show. Magic walked over to the couch while the crowd continued its vocal support. The chant continued for nearly three straight minutes, with Magic even feigning calling a time-out. Magic continued to smile, but his eyes belied his effervescent attitude. Deep inside himself, he was feeling something else.

The days and weeks before had been an emotional and physical blur. On September 24, Magic had married his longtime girlfriend Cookie, whom he began dating years earlier at Michigan State. The next month, they took a honeymoon to France as part of a Lakers team trip. They were in Paris for an exhibition game. Everyone, including the young couple, enjoyed the City of Light and was reticent to leave. Magic and Cookie wished they could spend more time walking hand in hand along the old cobblestone streets, but the team had to fly back home to finish up the preseason. By the time the team landed in Salt Lake City for their next game, Magic had an odd feeling well up inside him. He noticed he felt more tired than normal. Both he and those around him just chalked it up to jet lag. After all, it was a whirlwind trip back and forth across the entire Atlantic Ocean and then nearly the entire the United States. The NBA superstar asked for a few days off to recover before the official season began, but the team informed him he had to play at least a few minutes of the game. The Utah Jazz had a big-name duo in Karl Malone and John Stockton, and the fans wanted to see Magic on the court with them. Reluctant but agreeable, he went to the hotel and took a nap to get ready.

The phone rang in his room and woke him up with a start. It was the team's and his personal physician. Magic, he said, you have to come home right away. He didn't say much more than that. Still confused, Magic headed back to Los Angeles only a few hours after landing in Salt Lake City. His teammates noticed his absence but assumed he was pulling a veteran move of feigning an injury to get some more days of preseason rest. His team told the media he had the flu. His agent met him at LAX, and they drove to El Segundo to meet with Dr. Michael Mellman. The team had recently taken out a life insurance policy on Magic to cover a 3-million-dollar loan they had given him. The Lakers were notified via letter that the purchase was rejected on medical reasons but had been offered no specifics. Magic requested an explanation, and the next morning, Mellman received a Fedex envelope with the screening test results. In a small office later that day, Mellman asked Magic to sit down. He pulled out the FedEx envelope, removed the papers inside, and explained to Magic that he had tested positive for the HIV virus. All Magic heard was a death sentence.

Magic called his wife, who in a crazy twist of fate happened to be recently pregnant. Their relationship was often defined by Magic's desire to be in the spotlight and her desire for privacy. He did his thing "out there" and then returned home to her. Knowing he had a game to play, she was shocked to hear from him, but he said he would be home soon to explain. Since they had an on-again, off-again relationship before marriage, her first thought was he wanted a divorce. But she swallowed it down. Then, knowing he had recently visited his doctor, she asked him, "What's wrong, do you have AIDS or something?"

He didn't respond. Driving home, Magic recalled, he had faced many challenges in his life, including battling both Larry Bird and Michael Jordan on the basketball court. And yet, the hardest thing he ever did was that drive home to tell his wife he was HIV positive. He had broken off their marriage engagement twice, and almost a third time. Finally, they married, and now two months later, he was about to unload this devastating news on her.

He pulled into their driveway and paused in the car to collect himself. He finally mustered up the courage to walk into their house and quickly broke the news to her. He understood it was a terrible situation and he would leave if she wanted him to. Her answer was to put his hand on her belly where their child was growing and reassure him they would fight this thing together. Then they got down on their knees, the towering basketball superstar next to his shy, pregnant wife, and prayed for a miracle. Later that night, Johnson quietly walked into a bathroom in their house, closed the door, and began to call the long list of women he had unprotected sex with. As an NBA star, he had his pick of women. And these were "quality" women, not the kind that would have had HIV, he and the other players had told themselves.

For two weeks after, Magic did not play in a single game. The media was told he had the flu the whole time. He assured everyone he would be back soon but wanted to make sure to get some practice time in before playing. He didn't want to go back too quickly and injure himself after having had some time off. Meanwhile, the real story was that Magic and his doctor were waiting for confirmatory test results. Soon after, the nation's top HIV doctor confirmed the scary truth. There was no doubt Magic Johnson was HIV positive, and not only that, but it was already taking a toll on his immune system. He was told he could no longer play professional basketball. Even worse, his life might be over soon. The only good news he heard that day was that his wife, and therefore his baby, were HIV negative.

Magic asked his agent and good friend Lon Rosen to call his close friends Michael Jordan, Larry Bird, longtime Lakers Coach Pat Riley, and actor-comedian Arsenio Hall to break the news. They were devastated. Magic himself spoke directly to his parents and to his first son from a previous relationship who, at the time, was 10 years old. Andre was pulled out of school and brought home so he could speak to his father on the living room phone. Magic and Cookie decided they would then make a public announcement on Friday November 8, 1991.

On Thursday November 7, Lon got a call from a reporter at *USA Today*. They were being told Magic Johnson had HIV and would be retiring from the NBA. This was one day before Magic had been prepared to tell the news on his own terms. Faced with the story breaking ahead of the news conference, Magic decided to do the press conference right away. The Lakers were at Loyola Marymount University when an announcement came to stop practicing and head to the Forum right away. Once everyone arrived in the locker room, Magic quieted everybody and told his teammates what had unfolded. After a few minutes, he gathered himself and strode straight out to the podium, still smiling on the outside as he always did. In a firm voice, he broke the devastating news to the world: "Because of the HIV virus that I have attained, I will have to retire from the Lakers today".

The next night is when Magic found himself on the Arsenio Hall Show. After the crowd quieted down, he took a seat on the set's gray suede couch. Arsenio himself sat perched like a bird on a chair next to him. It was at that moment that Magic began what would become his lifelong journey. He became the face of the HIV virus. "I want everyone to practice safe sex and use condoms. I want to educate the public." Magic continued, "We don't have to run from it. We don't have to be ashamed of it. We have to make people aware of what's happening." Most important, he said we have to educate the black community.

At the time, little was known about HIV, and to most people, it was a disease that struck homosexuals. To address that line of thinking, Magic stated unequivocally, "I am far from being a homosexual. You know that." Perhaps out of nerves, or perhaps out of a desire to see him more as a victim of circumstance, the audience cheered. For society at large, someone who was lesbian/gay/bisexual stricken with HIV was less deserving of empathy, while in contrast a heterosexual was seen more as a "victim" of the disease. But to classify HIV as a "homo-sexual" disease, Magic stated, "That's so wrong." "Heterosexuals," he warned, "it's coming fast and we're going to have to prepare for it."

Despite the public support for Magic, privately he and his family continued to struggle socially. Restaurants where he had a table anytime he wanted no longer wanted him to dine there. Comedians who had been his friends began to make jokes about him onstage. His brother had to take time off from his job because of his coworkers. Even his 10-year-old son noticed that the other kids and adults around him were acting differently. Magic needed a direction. As an athlete, he needed to focus himself on a goal. Most of all, he needed guidance, so he sought out someone in his Hollywood circle he knew was fighting the AIDS disease.

Elizabeth Glaser was the wife of Starsky and Hutch star Paul Michael Glaser. She had contracted the HIV virus through a contaminated blood transfusion while giving birth. Unlike Cookie Johnson, Elizabeth's child was not spared, as Elizabeth had transferred the disease to her daughter through breastfeeding. Sadly, her child died from AIDS-related complications. Despite the tragic hand she was dealt, she continued to be a strong and inspiring woman. During their meeting, she asked Magic to be the face of the disease—a conduit of education. Johnson agreed to proudly take on the mantle. First, he tried working on policy with President George Bush but found it too difficult. So, he quit the president's council and instead turned to what he knew best—drawing people in through the television camera.

Sitting on a purple sofa, surrounded by children, Magic hosted a memorable Nickelodeon special. In "A Conversation with Magic Johnson," he talked with two young girls infected with HIV. In a clearly emotional moment, the girls told the world they only wished to be treated like everyone else. "I want people to know," 7-year-old and future HIV activist Hydeia Broadbent sniffled through tears, "that we're just normal people." "Aww, you don't have to cry," the gigantic Johnson reassured both the girl and the world, "because we are normal people."

A few weeks prior to the special airing, in an interesting twist of fate, it turned out Magic Johnson's name was still on the NBA All-Star ballot. He was still an eligible player. United in their love of the great Laker, fans across the nation voted him into the game. The game itself was slated to be played in a city known for its own magic, Orlando, Florida, the home of Walt Disney's "Magic" Kingdom. It couldn't have been a better screenplay. But as the game drew nearer, and the reality of Magic playing became apparent, suddenly without warning, attitudes within the league began to change. As a "victim," Magic had many of the players' public support. But as someone who might play an actual game against them, some NBA superstars bristled at the perceived threat to their health. Even the top of the NBA leadership had official meetings to decide if they wanted to "align" with Earvin Johnson. To their credit, NBA officials sought out the expertise of HIV scientific leaders, who assuaged their fears about Magic playing or passing on the disease. Armed with a better education, the NBA gave Magic the green light and welcomed him back for the 1992 NBA All-Star Game. The game started with many of the players hugging Magic, showing no fear of physical contact. Then, following the opening tip-off, the Magic show began. Johnson showed the world he still had it, even thrilling the crowd by going one-on-one with Michael Jordan. In what was the cherry on top of a perfect night, Magic made the last shot to win the game for the West, a moment that earned him MVP honors.

His comeback story didn't stop in Orlando. The Magic rebound tour then headed to Barcelona, where he captained the first-ever basketball Olympic Dream Team to a dominating gold medal. Fresh off yet another historic moment, Magic and the NBA prepared for him to return to play the next season. He was cleared by his doctors and ready to don a Lakers jersey once again. As a precaution, the NBA implemented new infection control procedures, especially for bleeding. It seemed like everything was back in line for Magic Johnson. But soon the storybook ending faded into reality, and the vocal opposition started again. This time, the most notable voice came from Magic's former Dream Team teammate Karl Malone. In his mind, Malone protested, he couldn't play as hard as he wanted to. He was a physical player, and bumps and bruises were an every-game experience. How could he do that with Magic Johnson on the court?

It all came to a head before the season even started. During a pre-season game in North Carolina, Johnson suffered a small cut on his arm and went over to his team's bench. Magic was used to having all the eyes in the house on him, but this time it was clear it was for a different reason. He could hear the murmurs in the crowd. He could see the fear in the other players' faces. Sensing the atmosphere, the longtime loyal Lakers athletic trainer chose to minimize the moment by not donning latex gloves. Instead, the lack of protection seemed even more shocking to everyone watching. In an effort to preserve the game and minimize the circus, Magic decided then he would leave the hardwood as a player and focus instead on spreading education within the minority community. He would have a short stint of a second comeback but decided he would leave the game this time on his own terms. Magic first entered the NBA spotlight as a rookie helping the Lakers to win an NBA championship by playing all five positions in Game 6 under Paul Westhead (Hank Gathers's future Loyola Marymount coach). Four more championships later, he would leave basketball the way he came in, with his head held high and that ever-present smile on his face.

There is no doubt that Magic Johnson's Announcement helped pave the way for people to reconsider who was at risk for the HIV virus. At the time, the disease was seen by many as a plague of the lesbian/gay/bisexual community. This narrative drew a social distinction between the "innocent" heterosexual victims versus the "guilty" lesbian/gay/bisexual or IV drug abuser. Magic himself had to dispel rumors of his own sexuality, even among his close friends in the NBA. He even admitted it was one of the reasons a wedge was driven between him and his longtime friend and NBA colleague Isiah Thomas. Magic believed Isiah had spread rumors about his sexuality and, as a result, lobbied to keep the future Hall of Famer off the 1992 Dream Team. The rift was so deep that the two men would not bury the hatchet until

2017, when, in an emotional moment during a televised interview, they finally hugged each other.

Magic's announcement wasn't just a big news story. It was actually a significant inflection point within the epidemiological research of HIV. As a result, there is a large amount of scientific literature dedicated just to studying trends after his announcement. It has even been dubbed the "Magic effect." Broadly, the Magic effect has been credited with helping bring national attention in the media to the HIV and AIDS crisis. The CDC reported that following the media coverage of Magic's HIV status, the average number of calls to its AIDS hotlines went from 4,000 per day to over 25,000 per day. Magic's infection helped reshape ethnic, social, and cultural beliefs about who was at risk for HIV. It also helped to differentiate between HIV as a disease that causes AIDS and the devastating effect of AIDS itself. Just to clarify, HIV is the virus that infects T-cells (CD-4 cells specifically) that are part of the body's immune system. AIDS is a syndrome that occurs once T-cell levels drop below a certain number. Someone can have HIV, but they don't develop AIDS unless the disease advances far enough to kill off a significant number of T-cells. As the combination of a professional basketball player, an African American, a wealthy individual, and a married heterosexual, Johnson represented an individual who had achieved the "American Dream." He also represented an eye-opening example for a population of individuals who may not have previously considered themselves at risk for HIV infection.

One effect many researchers have been able to demonstrate is that, following Magic's announcement, there was a significant increase in people undergoing HIV testing. The impetus to get tested for HIV was apparent both in males and females, spiking right after Magic's announcement. On the next page is a graph that depicts the number of testing submissions before and after Magic's announcement. They had already been collecting data when his announcement occurred around weeks 44–45. You can see the major change before and after his disclosure by both males and females.

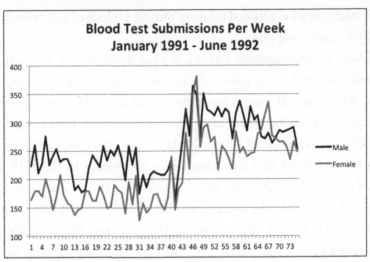

Male versus Female Blood Test Submission. Data Courtesy of James M. Tesoriero, PhD.

If you break the data down by age, you can see that the younger groups were more interested in getting tested than the older groups. The greatest total number and greatest spike of HIV testing was for people under 30 years old.

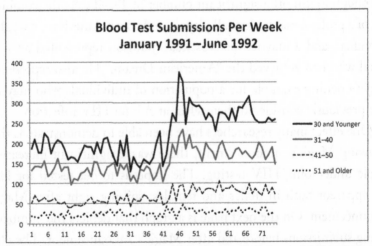

Blood Test Submissions by Age. Data Courtesy of James M. Tesoriero, PhD.

If we now look at testing rates for just African American and Hispanic people, there is still a spike after the announcement. But having separated out the two different groups, the spike for the black individuals studied turns out to be much higher than that for the Hispanic individuals studied. However, the spike effect actually dwindled rather quickly for both groups over a period of weeks. Here is the graph of the weekly test submissions before and after the announcement:

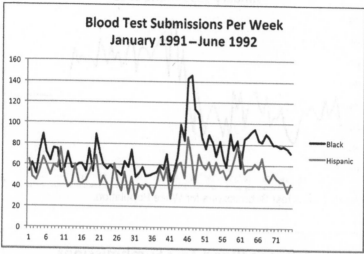

Weekly Blood Test Submissions for Black and Hispanic Populations.

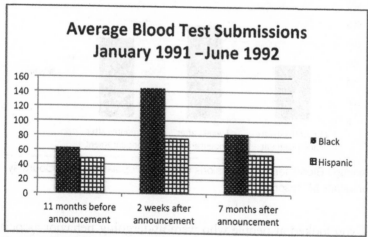

Average Blood Test Submissions for Black and Hispanic Populations. Data Courtesy of James M. Tesoriero, PhD.

Looking at the white population, the spike is also there. But unlike other racial/ethnic groups tested, the increased testing levels continued for another 20 or so months until the end of the study:

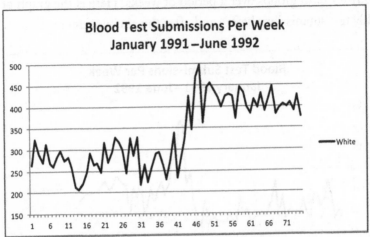

Weekly Blood Test Submissions for White Population.

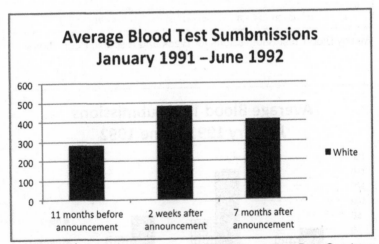

Average Blood Tests Submissions for White Population. Data Courtesy of James M. Tesoriero, PhD.

If you looked at people who were undergoing behavior associated with increased HIV transmission, the spike really only stands out for those individuals who admitted to having risky sexual partners. There was no real change in testing levels of persons who inject drugs or self-identified lesbian/gay/bisexual individuals. This is not that surprising given Magic's adamant message that his infection occurred via heterosexual transmission. If you look at the second group of graphs, you will also see a clear spike in the heterosexual group that likely occurred because his announcement seemed more targeted to them.

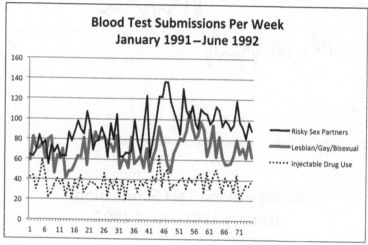

Weekly Blood Test Submissions for At-Risk Groups.

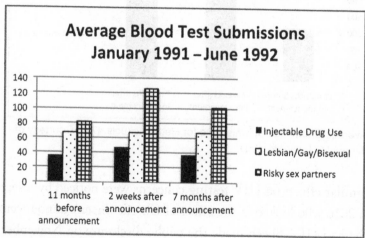

Average Blood Test Submissions for At-Risk Groups. Data Courtesy of James M. Tesoriero, PhD.

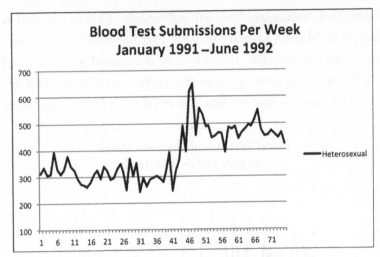

Weekly Blood Test Submissions for Heterosexuals.

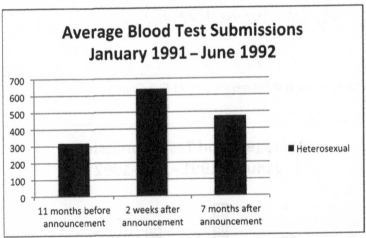

Average Blood Test Submissions for Heterosexuals. Data Courtesy of James M. Tesoriero, PhD.

Similar effects on HIV testing concerns were noticed by researchers in 2016 who looked at the effect of Charlie Sheen's announcement that he had HIV. Sheen made the public disclosure on November 17, 2015, almost 24 years to the day after Magic Johnson's. The authors of a study published in *JAMA Internal Medicine* found that Sheen's announcement corresponded with the greatest number of HIV-related

Google searches ever recorded in the United States. Only hours after the actor's announcement, searches related to HIV symptoms were 540 percent higher than usual. Searches related to HIV testing were 214 percent higher. But interestingly, searches related to condoms were only 72 percent higher. The lower condom search doesn't translate into anything definitive, but it is a similar trend, as with Magic, that HIV testing is more of a concern than condom use, at least by the parameters we can measure. As for the media coverage, Sheen's announcement corresponded with a 265 percent increase in HIV-related news stories. The authors of the article were encouraged by the results and emphasized that these celebrity disclosures and media coverage are moments where public health officials can capitalize on messaging in an organic way.

Beyond looking at just testing rates, at least thirteen studies have examined the impact of Magic's announcement on people's perceptions of vulnerability, or how worried someone is about contracting HIV. If you look at these studies as a whole, as a study in the *Journal of Health Communication* did in 2003, the average effect was essentially zero. But, if you break things down by age group, a pattern begins to emerge. For adults over the age of 18, the Magic effect seemed to increase feelings of vulnerability, while for those under 18, it seemed to have less of an effect. So what that means is that there was actually a negative effect on children. After the announcement, the fear of having HIV actually went down in the under-18 population. On the surface, this may seem like a bad thing, but authors of one study that looked at sixth- and eight-grade students in Boston pointed out that the children saw HIV as an "adult" disease. Therefore, their fear of contracting HIV through social contact went down, as it should. The children weren't necessarily thinking of it as a "sexual" disease. What's also interesting to note, though, is that the girls in the study were more prone to discussing the use of condoms, whereas the boys didn't seem to gravitate to that idea.

There was also a difference in how the boys and girls saw Magic Johnson six months after his announcement. The boys could better identify with him, whereas the girls saw him as a rich and famous person and not someone they could easily identify with. The girls also saw him as a less reliable source of information for AIDS and believed that there were likely people suffering with HIV/AIDS more than Magic was. This is in contrast to adults who increased their awareness of HIV as a *sexually-transmitted* disease and therefore realized *they* might be at more risk in their sexual relationships. If you combine the above narrative, you have Magic's message being lost on young girls, even though that same group is the one more willing to talk about condom use.

This difference in responsiveness to Magic's announcement between boys and girls was also highlighted in another study of 181 adolescents in four cities scattered in the North and Northeastern US. They came from Bangor and Portland, Maine; Boston, Massachusetts; and Madison, Wisconsin. The authors found that while age had no effect on message responsiveness, ethnicity did. Black adolescents were more likely to report increased AIDS awareness following Magic's announcement. Furthermore, females were more likely to report increased resistance to peer pressure to engage in sexual intercourse. In essence, Magic's effect was to empower female adolescents to resist peer pressure. This begins to shed light on what the cobra may have hid from most people looking on the surface of things. While everyone was looking at Magic, the cobra was eyeing his spouse, Cookie Johnson. Most people assumed Magic's message would resonate the most with young black men like himself, but perhaps it is the effect on young black women we should be looking more into.

Researchers from the New York Department of Health took an in-depth look at HIV counseling services following Magic's public disclosure. Initially, they saw the data that were previously described above, namely, the greatest increase in anonymous HIV testing was predominantly by white, heterosexual males under the age of 40 years old. Interestingly, the researchers said, the percentage of positive HIV tests dropped as the number of tests increased, suggesting that those seeking anonymous testing were possibly of lower risk, or at least weren't infected. So the great increase in testing was by those not infected with HIV. Which is good that the vast majority of people were unaffected, but it didn't seem to be identifying more cases simply by testing more people. Now, if you go back and look at that first graph of male versus female testing and examine it closely, you will see the greatest magnitude of the spike was actually female, and not male. Thus, the greatest surge in those seeking HIV testing right after Magic's November announcement was in the female population.

Further analysis was then conducted on women in New York State's Prenatal Care Assistance Program. This program offers women counseling and testing services during their pregnancies. When the numbers were run looking at the percentage of women in the program who agreed to HIV testing, the greatest Magic effect of all was filtered out. In the 10 months prior to the announcement, fewer than half (only 46 percent) of women agreed to be tested. This is in stark contrast to the nearly three-quarters (71 percent) of women who agreed to testing over the seven-month period after Magic's Forum press conference. The authors therefore proposed that maybe pregnant women were the most affected by Magic's televised disclosure. In fact, to see a pregnant woman and her growing child at risk of HIV, you only had to look to the left of Magic Johnson standing at the podium. Perhaps that very same day the Magic effect started to grow, off to the side in that very same room, there was a growing "Cookie Johnson effect."

These same authors also suggested another Cobra-like effect. Following Magic's announcement, it seemed that most of the people coming forward to be tested were low-risk individuals. As we have seen, most of the testing did not identify HIV-positive individuals. As a result, valuable resources were used for a group that may have needed them less. Perhaps the resources should be directed toward higher-risk groups such as Hispanics. The Hispanic population had the lowest response to Magic Johnson and yet at the time had the highest rate of positive tests. A 1990 study around the same time also showed that Hispanics considered sports figures to be the least credible source of

HIV/AIDS information. On the other hand, individuals who were in closer contact with the disease such as a physician, counselor, or patient were overwhelmingly perceived as the most credible sources of information. A proposed solution to this Cobra Effect of high versus low risk entailed training HIV/AIDS hotline operators to triage those callers by high versus low risk and simply educating those who are at low risk. Then for high-risk callers, operators could schedule testing. This certainly makes financial sense. Then again, the authors say, with that same increased wave of testing, there were at least 70 cases of HIV identified in New York. That's 70-plus people who hadn't known they were infected until that day thanks to the test.

Many researchers in the world of epidemiology, however, are quick to point out that attitudes and actions are not necessarily fully aligned. Although important, the variables we have looked at so far—resonating messages, education, increased testing, and vulnerability perceptions—may not be the most significant factor. In one quite serendipitous study, the risk behaviors of patients at a Maryland STD clinic were already being studied, when, suddenly, halfway through the 29-week study, the media was ablaze with the Magic Johnson story. Investigators quickly took advantage of this pivotal moment and analyzed the survey results before and after The Announcement. What they found was not great overall. At first, it looked like, almost across the board, risky behavior for most patients did not change. But first we should caution ourselves, since these results relied on asking patients to recall things over a 3-month period. This kind of research is subject to something statisticians like to refer to as a "recall bias." In other words, people being surveyed about the past either don't remember things accurately or may not be fully truthful in their responses. So, accepting that as a limitation, the researchers decided to delve deeper.

First, they looked at condom use before and after Magic's press conference. They found no difference with people who had steady or non-steady sex partners, as you can see in the table below. The percentages of each group are in parentheses:

Behavior	Preannouncement period[†]			Postannouncement period[§]			Chi-square	p value
	No. surveyed	Reporting behavior No.	(%)	No. surveyed	Reporting behavior No.	(%)		
Never used a condom during vaginal sex With steady sex partner(s)	144	60	(42)	73	39	(53)	2.7	0.10
With nonsteady sex partner(s)	102	24	(24)	48	11	(23)	0.0	0.93

Source: *Morbidity and Mortality Weekly Report*, Vol. 42, No. 3 (January 29, 1993), pp. 45–48.

They then looked at the effect the announcement had on risky "one-night stands." These data were more promising. It showed a reduction by 11 percent, which statistically speaking was significant.

Behavior	Preannouncement period[†]			Postannouncement period[§]			Chi-square	p value
	No. surveyed	Reporting behavior No.	(%)	No. surveyed	Reporting behavior No.	(%)		
Never used a condom during vaginal sex With steady sex partner(s)	144	60	(42)	73	39	(53)	2.7	0.10
With nonsteady sex partner(s)	102	24	(24)	48	11	(23)	0.0	0.93
Had "one-night stand(s)"	185	57	(31)	97	19	(20)	4.1	0.04

Source: *Morbidity and Mortality Weekly Report*, Vol. 42, No. 3 (January 29, 1993), pp. 45–48.

Finally, they looked at whether the risky behavior of having three or more sexual partners at a time changed following the November day. They found that there also was a statistically significant drop by 11 percent. Their data are in the last row of the table below:

Behavior	Preannouncement period[†]			Postannouncement period[§]			Chi-square	p value
	No. surveyed	Reporting behavior No.	(%)	No. surveyed	Reporting behavior No.	(%)		
Never used a condom during vaginal sex With steady sex partner(s)	144	60	(42)	73	39	(53)	2.7	0.10
With nonsteady sex partner(s)	102	24	(24)	48	11	(23)	0.0	0.93
Had "one-night stand(s)"	185	57	(31)	97	19	(20)	4.1	0.04
Had ≥3 sex partners of the opposite sex	186	60	(32)	97	20	(21)	4.2	0.04

[*] During the 3 months preceding the interview.
[†] From July 29, 1991, through November 1, 1991.
[§] From November 11, 1991, through February 14, 1992.

Source: *Morbidity and Mortality Weekly Report*, Vol. 42, No. 3 (January 29, 1993), pp. 45–48.

Intrigued by this finding, the researchers broke up the behavioral change by age groups, and what they found was a drop in all groups, except in 16-to-24-year-olds. In this group, there appears to even be a slight increase in risky behavior of multiple partners at a time following the announcement. Of course, there is another bias here in whom they are able to interview in an STD clinic, something called a "selection bias."

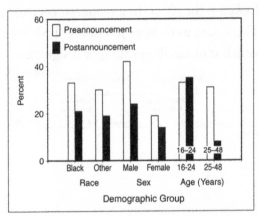

Percentage of sexually transmitted disease clinic patients who reported having had sex with three or more partners of the opposite sex during the 3 months preceding the interview, by race, sex, and age group and by response during the 14-week period before and after Earvin "Magic" Johnson's HIV-infection announcement on November 7, 1991. Source: *Morbidity and Mortality Weekly Report*, Vol. 42, No. 3 (January 29, 1993), pp. 45–48.

Another study taken in that same approximate age group took advantage of the captive audience provided by a class of rural, Midwestern university psychology students. A survey was given to the students before and after Magic's announcement in exchange for extra credit. Answers from the semester before the announcement versus the semester after were gathered and analyzed. There were no differences in attitudes or perceived personal risk of HIV before versus after the announcement. A range of 83 to 89 percent of the college students felt that they were at little or no risk of HIV infection. More than half (52.6 percent) reported that Magic's disclosure did not change their sexual behavior. Fewer than half (47.4 percent) reported that it did have an impact on their sexual behavior. When the authors then looked at those psychology students who said Magic did have an effect on their sexual behavior versus those who said they did not change their behavior, they actually found no difference in percentages of condom use or number of sexual partners. So, while there was a perceived change in behavior, there wasn't really a difference in the rates of actual risky behavior. The authors of the study hypothesized that while Magic's disclosure had a subjective emotional effect prompting a resolution to change, it did not lead to actual measurable behavioral changes.

It's now almost three decades later, and the actual effect of Magic Johnson's very public announcement is difficult to assess. Like any celebrity, whether it be Charlie Sheen's HIV status or Angelina Jolie's breast cancer gene, a marked interest in the public occurs anytime we can put a face on an issue. Still, like a new year's resolution or the waning interest in news cycles, prolonged behavioral changes are hard to maintain. Today, there are about 37 million people living with HIV across the globe. In 2017, almost 2 million people became newly infected with HIV. Almost 40,000 were living in the United States, and 10 percent were black women.

Below is a chart from 2017 showing new HIV diagnoses in the United States. Keep in mind that in 1992, the year after Magic found out his diagnosis, AIDS had become the number-one killer of men, especially black men, between the ages of 25 and 44. It was the second-

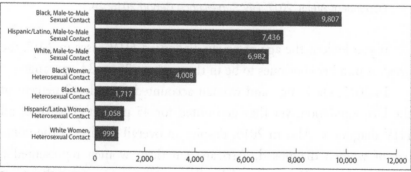

Source: CDC. Diagnoses of HIV Infection in the United States and Dependent Areas, 2017. *HIV Surveillance Report 2018*; 29.

leading cause of death for black women in the same age group. The graph below is now 25 years later.

If you look at the group that's right in the middle, you find heterosexual black women. To the right are groups with male-male or female-female sexual contact, and we have seen Magic's announcement was not directed at nor did it affect this self-identifying population. If you look to the left of the graph, you see black heterosexual men, who were thought to most identify with Magic. Therefore, the group that seems to be the closest to Magic and Cookie Johnson's demographic and in need of HIV intervention are black heterosexual women.

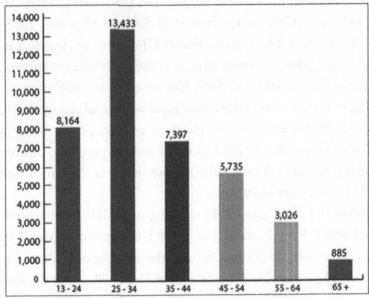

Source: CDC. Diagnoses of HIV Infection in the United States and Dependent Areas, 2017. *HIV Surveillance Report* 2018; 29.

If you look at the age of newly diagnosed HIV cases in 2017, the greatest number continues to be in the younger 25-to-34 age range.

In 2015, black men and women accounted for only 12 percent of the US population, yet they accounted for 45 percent (17,670) of all HIV diagnoses. Also in 2015, despite an overall decline in the number of women diagnosed, African American women represented a disproportionate 61 percent of the diagnoses among women that year.

Despite the promising fact that infection rates are trending downward, black women are still diagnosed with HIV at a rate 16 times higher than white women in the United States.

Below is a graph showing the trend of HIV Diagnoses among Women by Race/Ethnicity from 2005 to 2014. You can see significant progress has been made in the black female category running along the top of the graph, but the black female group is still significantly more

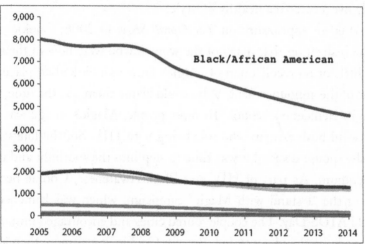

Number of HIV Diagnoses among Women by Race/Ethnicity. Source: CDC Fact Sheet, Trends in US HIV Diagnoses Among Women, 2005–2014, February 2016.

affected than other ethnicities.

The good news is that since the introduction of antiretroviral therapy, the fight against the epidemic of HIV and AIDS has seen great progress. Today, scientists have even identified a potential prophylactic benefit of taking HIV drugs 72 hours after exposure (PEP = postexposure prophylaxis). But, the disease is far from vanquished, and certain demographics continue to struggle in the battle more than others. When Magic made his announcement in 1991, it was clearly intended to target black heterosexual men, but perhaps the target that also should have been aimed at was African American women. Maybe, like Magic himself felt on that difficult drive home, things were more concerning where his own wife and baby were concerned.

For 15 years, from 1990 to 2005, the number of AIDS-related deaths increased and reached a peak in 2004. During this time, Cookie Johnson continued to stand more in the background while her husband, the consummate public speaker, continued to be the face of HIV. His face, however, remained vibrant and strong. Some people even questioned whether he actually had HIV. Others pointed out that Magic was rich and famous and had his pick of doctors, medicine, and could easily live a care-free healthy lifestyle.

After an appearance on *The Oprah Show* in 2006, Cookie came to the realization that many of the women who were now in their 20s had little or no recollection of Magic's fame as a basketball player, let alone of the announcement. Who could blame them? At the time, they were in elementary school. To most people, Magic's image was of a successful businessman who was living with HIV. So, the longstanding shy spouse decided it was time to step into the spotlight and up to the podium. As part of HIV and Black Awareness, Cookie became part of the "I stand with Magic" campaign, which was launched on World AIDS Day. The couple toured cities and encouraged minorities to get educated and get tested. But, for Cookie, it was more than about just encouraging testing. She wanted to share what she learned about HIV/AIDS with other women, who might be going through a situation similar to her own. This time, the target moved closer to African American females.

There is no doubt the celebrity effect is real. Magic Johnson, Charlie Sheen, and Angelina Jolie all showed their public announcements could be used as a priming effect to encourage testing and helped promote consistent messaging in the media.

The journey of Magic Johnson is the journey of the HIV virus in society—from fear of the unknown to acceptance. Today, thanks to ground-breaking discoveries in medicine, people can now think of HIV as a chronic illness such as diabetes and not a death sentence. Even so, it is still a preventable disease that kills millions of people. It should still be feared. Just because Magic Johnson's smiling face shines down from a billboard in Hollywood does not mean young black men and women should ignore the practices of safe sex. It also took 15 years for the spotlight to widen and shine on a significantly vulnerable HIV community, namely young African American women. Magic Johnson and his foundation continue to be rightfully lauded for all they have done, but maybe making Magic Johnson the sole beaming face of the announcement and subsequent campaign has had some unintended effects. Scientific research has shown that Magic was successful in raising awareness and changing attitudes in a critical time, but did society miss out on actually affecting behavioral change? Did the Cobra Effect allow attitudes to change but prevent actual action? And did we ignore an especially important demographic that was shielded in the shadows by the Cobra Snake? As Magic himself has said, he is both the blessing and the curse of the HIV virus.

3

Lyle Alzado and the Steroid Conversation

THE BLACK MARKET IS A real thing. It exists wherever unregulated transactions in the world occur. It is not a single website on the nefarious Dark Web or a distant flea market in Bangladesh spotted with Turkish rugs and Russian tanks. It is a concept that can be traced and studied. It even has a slang term. To those in the know, the black market is called "System D," a term that comes from French-speaking Africa and the Caribbean where motivated and resourceful entrepreneurs are called "débrouillards." The System D economy is impossible to fully capture from a numbers perspective, but economists have tried multiple times. In a 2006 report, Friedrich Schneider calculated that the worldwide black market was worth almost $10 trillion. Just to put this into perspective, the entire United States GDP is close to $14 trillion.

In order to study and analyze it, Schneider, an economics professor at Johannes Kepler University in Austria, took on the difficult task of first defining the shadow economy. Since it is an unregulated and nebulous system, setting boundaries and rules upon it is a challenge in itself. He defined the shadow economy as "unreported income from the production of legal goods and services—either from monetary or barter transactions—and so includes all economic activities that would generally be taxable, were they reported to the tax authorities." Using that definition, he and his coauthors started by looking at models of the world economies and calculating causes and effects based on known variables. They then looked to see how things in real life differed from the theoretical model calculations. By doing this comparison, they could examine "unknown variables" like the black market. In the economics and statistics world, this is known as "MIMIC."

Using the "MIMIC" approach, Schneider and his group published data in 2018 showing a gradual decline in the shadow market. Here is a graph showing informal economies in various world regions as a percent of their GDP for various years from 1991 to 2015.

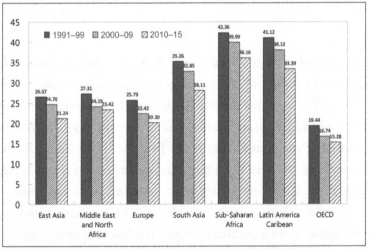

Shadow Economy by Region (average, percent of GDP).
Source: Courtesy of Leandro Medina and Friedrich Schneider

What we can determine from the graph is that there appears to be an overall decline in shadow markets, but they exist, and they are still thriving. We also may be underestimating their sizes as digital transactions become more and more common. So why do black markets exist in the first place? Some exist due to surplus and demand differences between neighboring economies. This is illustrated by smuggling cows from India to Bangladesh. In India, cows are considered sacred and preserved, whereas in Bangladesh they are slaughtered and sold for their meat. Others exist where cost and access to items are limited. Medical items are one such example, with perhaps the biggest black-market player being unregulated and possibly harmful Botox.

Government regulations can be a cause of a black market forming, as we saw with Prohibition and illegal alcohol sales in the United States. But there can also be unintended consequences of these regulations. By banning the sale and production of alcohol, for example, the control of illegal alcohol production fell to nefarious groups and further empowered them. Another unintended consequence of government regulation and black-market creation may be the lack of open and necessary communication.

A more recent example of this unintended lack of open and necessary communication can be found in the not-so-dark and seedy corners of the farmers' market. There, a black market of unpasteurized milk has sprung up. Nearly three decades ago, in response to increases in illnesses, the United States FDA banned the sale of raw milk across state lines. Most individual states followed suit and significantly limited its sale or banned it all together. There was always a slow trickle of shadow market sales of raw milk, but a resurgence seems to be occurring in response to new food movements, especially among younger generations. Some of these movements center around consumers moving closer to their food supply or limiting how much we change what Mother Nature naturally produces. And, as a result, pasteurization is sometimes seen as a blockade to fulfilling the tenets of this food ideology.

Pasteurization is a process named for the scientist Louis Pasteur, and before your eyes glaze over at any discussion deeper than the mere mention of it, what if someone told you the story of pasteurization is also the story of beer? Would that get your attention? Well, it's true. In the mid-1800s, Pasteur's scientific expertise was employed to determine why a certain type of beet-sugar-based alcohol was spoiling. The French biologist began by examining the liquid under a microscope and found that before it spoiled, the beer-like alcohol had mostly round and plump yeast organisms. But when it spoiled, these were mostly replaced by rod-shaped bacteria. It was these bacteria that were causing the beer to spoil. In fact, it appeared to Pasteur that this was the very same type of bacteria that was used to make vinegar. A culprit was found and needed to be eliminated.

In subsequent experiments, Pasteur fine-tuned a method of heating to kill the bacteria but save the beer. Successful in its defense of beer, this method was soon used to preserve wine and then brought out on a larger scale to kill the tuberculosis-causing bacteria in milk. Pasteur's method of pasteurization would eventually be further modernized into a high-temperature, short-time method known as HTST pasteurization. With this method, the harmful bacteria in milk can quickly and easily be killed. A side effect, though, is that some of the proteins in the milk are also affected by the high heat, and as the shape of the proteins change, so can the taste of the milk. This process both makes the milk safer to drink and can preserve its shelf life. Harmful bacteria like E. coli, Listeria, and salmonella are essentially destroyed. Opponents of this process, however, posit that the heating process also kills off beneficial microorganisms and enzymes that may be useful to the body. Advocates of raw milk say these key ingredients help produce stronger immune systems and promote better digestion.

In defense of pasteurization, the CDC and FDA can point toward some important statistics. In 1938, milk alone caused 25 percent of all outbreaks stemming from food- and water-related sickness. With the implementation of modern pasteurization techniques, that number would eventually fall to just 1 percent. Raw milk also has very little vitamin D. During the pasteurization process, this important vitamin can be added to the milk. Proponents of pasteurization also point to the unfortunate recent deaths of children related to raw milk consumption, particularly a toddler in Australia in 2014.

The raw-milk consumer camp has been able to circumvent the government's system in a number of ways. Some of them purchase what is called a cow-share, meaning they all pitch in to buy the cow and therefore are entitled to share the raw milk it produces for free. Others use a "buyers club" approach—made famous for delivery of HIV drugs during the AIDS epidemic. There are a handful of pet stores that market raw cow and goat milk for dogs, but it's not uncommon for humans to take it home and guzzle the milk themselves. The Amish have also gotten involved in this marketing and distribution of raw milk.

Raw milk advocates are quick to explain they don't always disagree with pasteurization as an option for consumers. It's the lack of communication and appropriate legislation for consumer demand that is their concern. If an individual wants to do something in which he or she understands the risks, like smoking cigarettes or drinking alcohol, then they should be allowed to do so. That may be acceptable for adults, some people will say, but the children are a different story. They may not be making these choices for themselves. In addition, not everyone who is buying raw milk may be aware of the possibility of higher disease risk.

While the CDC, the American Academy of Pediatrics, and the American Medical Association all strongly advise people not to drink raw milk, some states are starting to open the conversation up to new legislation. An estimated 3 percent of the population is consuming raw milk, and raw milk sales are legal, albeit with restrictions in about 30 states. This may make raw milk advocates a little happier, but choosing to drink raw milk is still not without measurable risks. According to the CDC, from 2007 to 2012, there were 81 outbreaks of illnesses attributed to raw milk consumption. That is compared to just an average of about three a year from 1993 to 2006. Some will point out, though, that a majority of these outbreaks involved severe diarrhea that may have come from milk tainted with feces bacteria and not from the milk bacteria itself.

Nevertheless, the raw milk black market continues to grow. What's needed to improve safety and regulation is an open and honest conversation. Simply labeling something as dangerous, imposing government regulations, and ignoring further conversations can backfire. This is where the Cobra Effect occurs. By ignoring the black market and those who wish to purchase from it, the conversation dies, and further harm may come to those the government was trying to protect.

SIMILARLY, WE HAVE SEEN THE unintended consequences of regulation and a subsequent lack of open and honest discussion with steroids in sports. Lyle Alzado, a former lineman for the Los Angeles Raiders, is one of the first US sports stars to admit to having used anabolic steroids and notably died at the young age of 43. His *New York Times* obituary on May 15, 1992, defined him as a "self-styled symbol of the dangers of steroid abuse".

Alzado is one of the most recognizable faces in the storied history of the NFL. Most of the time, he appeared with a grizzled beard jutting below a thick bush of black hair. If a child were asked to draw a picture of a barbarian, it would resemble Alzado. He was a two-time Pro Bowl defensive end in the NFL, a Defensive Player of the Year, and played in two Super Bowls. He was the centerpiece of a formidable Denver defense dubbed the "Orange Crush" after the color of their uniforms (and a soft drink). Later, he was a fellow renegade on the Raiders. He had a Super Bowl championship ring, which he was more than happy to show off at a trendy West Hollywood nightspot dubbed Alzado's. He was a larger-than-life character on the football field and on the big screen. His massive body became a physical barrier against the world. The bigger his biceps or chest, the easier it was to shield himself from his past and his insecurities.

Lyle's biography typically begins with the recitations that he was born the son of a Spanish-Italian father and a Jewish mother in Brooklyn. But this two-line epitaph was not Lyle Alzado. Lyle was born on the streets or, more specifically, in street fights. It was on the streets where Alzado's notorious "kill or be killed" mentality was forged. Fighting was in his blood. It was the backbone of his DNA. Lyle's father was a fighter. He was a former boxer who did not stop punching people even after he left the confines of the ring. Initially following in his father's footsteps, Lyle decided to try his hand at boxing. When he stepped between the ropes, technique was thrown out the door. His poignant strategy was to just "pound" the other guy. He was, as he admits, violent by nature. Despite his rawness, Lyle managed to put together a decent amateur boxing career, even losing a disputed contest for the Golden Gloves. But boxing wasn't where he wanted to dedicate his life. Lyle associated boxing with his father, and, as he put it, his father was not a good man. To anyone who knew the Alzado family, that was a scary understatement.

His sister called their childhood home a "house of horrors." His father was an abusive alcoholic who regularly beat his wife and children. Lyle saw himself as the protector, especially for his mother and sister. One particular day, when his father got out of his car to assault their mother, Lyle ran down the stairs and punched his father. The older man's jawbone broke from the force of the young man's fist. No stranger to a jail cell, Lyle's own father had his son arrested for assault. Lyle's rap sheet would continue to grow over the years, mirrored only by his anger and resentment. He sometimes wished he was born in an earlier time of gladiators. At least then he could unleash the hostility that boiled inside of him onto other people without ending up in prison. A hellfire grew in Lyle, and it was in football where he found an outlet.

Alzado's professional football career began when he took over for a man nicknamed "Tombstone." As a member of the Denver Broncos and one of the best defensive players in the National Football League, Alzado helped lead his team to the Super Bowl on January 15, 1978. The game took place in the New Orleans Superdome, and Alzado fought one of the toughest games of his life that day. But despite the top-notch performance by Alzado and the "Orange Crush" defense, the Broncos offense turned the ball over eight times. As a result, the Broncos were dominated most of the game by the Cowboys, and Lyle's dream of a Super Bowl ring were crushed. Dissatisfied with the outcome of the game and coming up short, something Lyle was not used to, Alzado briefly contemplated a career change to boxing. He tested the waters by competing in an eight-round exhibition match with legendary heavyweight champion Muhammad Ali. In typical but bizarre fashion, Alzado didn't back down from Ali and tried to make the show a real fight. Ali quickly reminded him what he did for a living and zapped him with a few well-placed jabs. By the next season, the relationship between Lyle and the Broncos organization had officially soured. Denver decided they no longer wanted him and traded him away. Lyle would have a brief stint with the Cleveland Browns but soon found his tribe and a career rebirth with the Los Angeles Raiders.

It was there in LA where Alzado's rage took center stage. He was nicknamed "Rainbow" for his mood swings, a "Human Volcano" because he was poised to erupt at any moment, "Three-Mile Lyle" after the nuclear meltdown, and "Darth Raider" after the ominous Star Wars character clad in all black. Alzado was seen as an antihero who described football not as fun, but as a war. At that time in 1982, the Raiders proudly carried the reputation of being a bunch of "tough, intimidating misfits." One NFL coach called the union between Alzado and the Raiders "the perfect marriage—the kind they make in hell." Al Davis, a team owner known for his unorthodox choices, decided to take a chance on a player who may have been past his prime, and yet, Alzado didn't slow down. In fact, he helped lead the piratical bunch to a Super Bowl Championship—a day that many who knew him called the one time in his life Lyle was finally happy.

Yet throughout all of his success, there always hung the cloud of "roid rage." Even as Alzado racked up the accolades, his bouts of anger and purported steroid abuse continued to haunt him. His temper flared on and off national television. In a 1982 Divisional playoff game, he ripped the helmet off New York Jets lineman Chris Ward and threw it at him, inspiring a rule specifically barring the act of taking a helmet off and using it as a weapon (the so-called "Alzado rule"). Off the field, Lyle chased a man who side-swiped his car through a neighborhood. On multiple occasions, he was reported to have pulled people out of their cars to beat them.

In one account, he was with his gym training partner John Romano driving his black Mercedes down a street that had two lanes going in both directions. Romano is a longtime bodybuilder with deep ties to the industry and insider knowledge of steroid use. Lyle was in the right-hand lane and another guy was trying to pass a car in the left lane. The driver quickly cut off Lyle in the right lane as the light in front of them suddenly turned red. Both men were forced to slam on their brakes. The man in the front car looked up and into his rearview mirror to the see "the most feared man in the NFL" getting out of the car behind him. Lyle approached the driver's side to confront the man. Before Romano knew what had happened, Lyle's hands were inside the driver's window. Lyle proceeded to drag the man out of his car and throw him up against its side. Romano yelled from the car, "Lyle c'mon." With his rage temporarily interrupted, Lyle looked around, made a comment to the other driver, and got back into his car.

Lyle and his anger were no stranger to domestic violence and divorce. In one heated confrontation, his wife tried to run him over with her car. Lyle managed to hold onto the hood of the speeding car throughout Manhattan Beach. This event was not long after he had dragged that same spouse out of a party to beat her. Lyle would have to check restaurants when he arrived to make sure no one there would set him off. And he yelled, all the time. He needed the steroids to be both physically and mentally strong, once writing, "I just didn't feel strong unless I was taking something."

Alzado's steroid abuse was no secret. He started using in college and continued even after his NFL retirement. A comment by a fan or former teammate that he wasn't as big as he used to be would lead him right back to the pills and needles. While a member of the Los Angeles Raiders, he worked closely with team physician Rob Huizenga on curbing the side effects but had no intention of stopping. In his book, *You're Okay, It's Just a Bruise*, Huizenga writes that he told Alzado his cholesterol and liver function were so abnormal from steroid abuse that he was "a heart attack waiting to happen." Alzado's behavior was described by the doctor as falling along a rainbow; some days he was "kind and considerate," and other days he was a "raging animal." When police would be called to his house following domestic violence incidents, he would transform back into Dr. Jekyll. He would calmly talk to the officers, and each time it would end the same way—with him signing autographs for the officers.

He was never taught how to love, nor could he ever fill the hole he felt in his heart. Physically he could get stronger, but emotionally he was always weak. He constantly strove for validation. When his team finally won the Super Bowl in 1984, amidst a throng of fans, players, and the media, Lyle, with his eyes wild, pulled a reporter he knew to the back simply to ask him how he played. The validation from the writer that he had played well meant everything to him. Even later, when he was a Hollywood magnet and a celebrity, he still needed his abusive father's approval. Once when he was visiting a friend in his old neighborhood, he spotted his father tailing him. Alzado turned his car around to confront the old man and stared him down, but even then his enormous frame wasn't enough to protect him. Panic took over, and in a cold sweat, the monstrous football player sped away, driving across a neighbor's lawn just to get around his father. Later, even after Alzado helped lead the Raiders to a Super Bowl victory, he decided to pay his father a visit to tell him about an award he was very proud to be receiving, which recognized him for his generous work with sick children. In fact, Lyle was well known for his charity time with children, often visiting children's hospitals after practice. He became a larger-than-life superhero and defender who gave them hope and encouragement at their bedside. When he finally did meet with his father to share the good news, all he got in return was a grunt and a request for money.

In the rise-and-fall saga of Lyle Alzado, his success is sometimes described as arising from a deal with the devil. As his childhood and best friend Marc Lyons saw it, one day the "devil came to collect." In 1990, when Alzado was marrying his fourth wife, something in him felt, and even looked, off. He walked down the aisle at their wedding, but it didn't look right. He had a stiff-legged, almost mechanical gait. The wide smile on his face belied the worry in his mind. The morning after, he was too tired to even drive. Later during the honeymoon, while signing autographs for some fans, he noticed a quizzical look on their faces. He looked down and what he saw shocked him. His iconic signature was now just a series of circles. Concerned, he went to see his former team doctor in Beverly Hills. The test results took a sledgehammer to the world he had built. He was diagnosed with primary brain lymphoma—a rare brain cancer.

His illness put a further financial strain on an already struggling newlywed couple. Lyle had already lost most of his money to previous divorces and failed business ventures. To cut expenses, they moved out of his million-dollar Palos Verdes mansion and into an apartment in Marina Del Rey. Shortly after the move, a business deal had fallen through, and a subpoena was issued for Alzado to appear in civil court. Per protocol, it was to be hand-delivered by a deputy marshal. This time, when the police showed up at his door, it didn't end up with him shaking hands and signing autographs. The banging on the apartment door woke Alzado up at 7 a.m. A weakened Alzado flung open the door in a rage. He tried to steady himself but lost his balance. He fell toward the 110-pound female officer at the entranceway. Seeing Alzado falling toward her, she reacted quickly to the perceived aggression and Maced him.

Over the next year, Alzado would undergo radiation treatment for the cancer growing in his brain. His body would waste away to a former shell of the mountainous man he used to be. He lost the rest of his hair. His cheeks sank in. His clothes no longer fit. Reminiscent of the Raiders logo, he even had to wear an eye patch for his vertigo. Finally, in a quest to absolve himself of his hidden guilt, he decided to tell the truth about his steroid abuse. In 1991, less than a year before his death, the former football player sat down for an interview with *Sports Illustrated* titled "I'm Sick and I'm Scared." In it, he apologizes for lying about his steroid abuse and documents his addiction.

He goes on to describe the drive in athletes that leads them to steroids and performance enhancing drugs (PEDs) and how pervasive the abuse really is:

> They are so intent on being successful that they're not concerned with anything else. No matter what an athlete tells you, I don't care who, don't believe them if they tell you these substances aren't widely used.

He estimated that ninety percent of the athletes he knew used anabolic steroids.

He also warns others about the dangers of steroids. On first read-through, it sounds like he is warning that something bad will happen to you physically if you abuse steroids. But, maybe his statements were more profound than he has been given credit for, since steroids can take a toll on your life in different ways whether it be run-ins with the law or a fractured relationship:

> Whoever is doing this stuff, if you stay on it too long or maybe if you get on it at all, you're going to get something bad from it.

Alzado and some doctors have attributed his years of steroid abuse as a risk factor for developing the brain tumor that ultimately led to his death. Others are quick to point out there is no direct connection between Alzado's condition and steroid abuse. Alzado also began using human growth hormone (HGH) during a failed NFL comeback as well as newer injectable testosterone that lasted two to four times longer in the body. HGH at that time had been sourced from cadavers, and there was medical evidence linking its use to harmful side effects, including transmission of a brain-eating disorder, Creutzfeldt-Jakob disease, the human equivalent of "mad cow" disease. Newer versions were genetically engineered to avoid the risk of human disease transmission, and these were not tested for in the NFL during the late 1980s. But in an age where media and fan approval can change at a whim, what's easiest for most people is to see Lyle's rise and fall as a morality tale. A fable where someone who abused drugs, bullied women, and regularly beat people up on his quest to the top died as a weak man in his early 40s. Even Alzado himself had a premonition he was living a life on borrowed time. He would die young one day, he said, just like Elvis.

For a long time, Alzado became the face of the fight against steroid use—but did he or the league do enough to change the perception of steroid use? In 1987, two years after Alzado's retirement, the NFL began testing players for steroids but did nothing to punish those who were caught using. And the next year, in the wake of the Ben Johnson

Olympic sprinting steroids fiasco, as part of the Anti-Drug Abuse Act of 1988 pushed by Senator Joe Biden, Congress made possession and distribution of anabolic steroids for nonmedical purposes a crime. Biden called it "cheating" and "absolutely un-American." Then in 1990, Congress passed the Anabolic Steroids Control Act that placed anabolic steroids in the same legal class as amphetamines, methamphetamines, opium, and morphine. Yet, the abuse in professional sports continued, and it was no longer just among football's best players.

In 1991, Major League Baseball's commissioner Fay Vincent, reacting to rumors of Jose Canseco's steroid abuse, sent a memo to all the baseball clubs prohibiting all drugs, including steroids. It was largely ignored. In fact, the memo had to be reissued by Commissioner Bud Selig a few years later in 1997, since the apathy or ignorance of the baseball managers still persisted. The next year, in 1998, sluggers Mark McGwire and Sammy Sosa dueled in an epic battle of home run kings amid rumors of steroid abuse. The league continued to turn a blind eye, as the home run race was restoring baseball fans' interest in the game. It wasn't until 2002, which was ten years after Alzado's death—and the year after Barry Bonds broke McGwire's home run record again amidst steroid abuse allegations—that Major League Baseball began formally testing players for steroids. Also at that time, federal authorities had launched an investigation into BALCO, a California lab that was suspected of selling performance-enhancing drugs to the elite athletes of several other sports.

One of the most visible users was Bill Romanowski, another legendary Denver Broncos defensive player known for his killer instinct who was being supplied designer steroids and human growth hormone. Like Alzado, Romanowski was known for his violent temper, which was not limited to pounding just the other team. In 2003, Romanowski attacked and injured one of his own teammates during a scrimmage. After a play, he ripped off the other player's helmet and then proceeded to fracture his orbital eye socket with a punch. The other player sued for damages of $3.4 million, arguing Romanowski was under the influence of "roid rage" when he attacked him. The argument was later rejected by the judge on the grounds he could not prove Romanowski had actually used steroids on the same day as the attack. Then, in 2005, nearly 35 years after Alzado entered the NFL, sparked by a book admission from baseball slugger Jose Canseco and media attention, six big-name Major League Baseball players, including home run kings Mark McGwire, Sammy Sosa, and Canseco himself, testified before Congress about drugs in baseball. Many of these players initially denied or deflected the questions on steroids only to later admit to or be exposed for having abused steroids and other PEDs during their careers. Nevertheless, none of these guys looked like Alzado's gaunt face on the cover of *Sports Illustrated*, and none of them were dying from cancer.

Perhaps the biggest community to reject Alzado's claims of the dangers of steroids was the one he was closest to—the bodybuilding community. At the time of his admission, steroids were everywhere. They were readily available in the gym, on the field, and in Hollywood. Gold's Gym in Venice had become a mecca for bodybuilding where, to the initiated, the priests gave out steroids like communion. There was even a class on steroid use in the back called "Sunday School." At the time, Gold's Gym might have been one the coolest places on Earth, where you could work out among some of the world's best athletes and biggest celebrities. Before Hollywood took an interest, bodybuilders were seen as bouncers, or bodyguards, or guys who broke legs for bookies. But once the celebrities joined in, bodybuilding's image softened and became a unique fraternity.

To bodybuilders, Gold's Gym was a brotherhood. Outside of the gym, you were a "freak" or "mutant"—someone dedicating his life to chasing a physique of 265 pounds and 3 percent body fat, which of course is not natural. But inside, you were among your people. You could be living in the parking lot, but once you walked through those gym doors, you were among family. There, the battle against Mother Nature and normalcy happened out in the open every day with barbells and dumbbells, and with a syringe. Steroids were no secret. They were part of the path. Even today, the sport of bodybuilding needs a separate division dedicated to being "drug-free."

To the gymgoers, everyone at Gold's was visible proof that steroids worked. As far as anyone knew, no one besides Lyle was dying of brain cancer from anabolic steroids. Even the doctors at the gym who prescribed the drugs and had them delivered to the front desk were using them. One doctor in particular, Dr. Walter Jekot, became the face of a growing movement to prescribe anabolic steroids to HIV patients. Jekot noticed that his HIV-positive patients who used steroids didn't appear to be succumbing to AIDS and their bodies weren't wasting away. In fact, many of them looked outwardly healthy and strong. So, in 1984, the West Los Angeles physician became the first of several doctors to prescribe anabolic steroids as a treatment for AIDS.

It is in this intersection that a rumor began to grow that still pervades the bodybuilding community and message boards. At the crossroads of drugs, bodybuilders, Hollywood nightlife, and HIV/AIDS in the 1980s, it wasn't hard to connect anyone in the close-knit group of steroid users in Los Angeles with someone who was lesbian/gay/bisexual. Even Jekot claimed during his own trial that former football player and drug dealer Barry Voorhees, whose client list included Lyle Alzado, offered him homosexual favors in exchange for steroids. And then there was the unsubstantiated whisper that Lyle Alzado would cruise Santa Monica Boulevard looking for boys. While this has been denied repeatedly by Lyle's own wives and family members, the rumor still slinks along the underbelly of the steroid world, especially because B-cell lymphoma of the brain was an AIDS disease. Lyle's initial diagnosis by the pathologist at UCLA was T-cell lymphoma, but in Oregon it was changed to B-cell lymphoma by the pathologist there. Plus, the conspiracy theorists say, Lyle had pneumonia before he died and AIDS-related pneumonia was a real thing. Never mind, they say, that the doctors in Oregon who treated him before his death "went overboard in AIDS testing" and found no evidence of the virus. The UCLA doctors tested for HTLV-3 (the AIDS virus) and HTLV-1 (which is an AIDS-related, lymphoma-causing virus) and found nothing. And his pneumonia was bacterial in origin, which can easily be related to chemotherapy's effects on the immune system and not from the organisms associated with AIDS. But to the bodybuilding community, it was a cover-up. In fact, when Lyle failed to make a comeback in the NFL at age 41, they couldn't believe it. There was no way the Superman of Gold's Gym couldn't have done it. Did they see the shape he was in during that Maria Shriver interview? He never looked better. (For the record, he absolutely denied using steroids in that same interview with Arnold Schwarzenegger's wife.) Anyway, speculators suggested he must have quit his comeback because of a secretly positive HIV test. But those who knew him adamantly denied that line of thinking. Alzado was let go by a savvy team owner because the grizzled veteran was now older and riddled with injuries.

So what are we to do then with the parable of Lyle Alzado? Can we learn any lessons from his abuse of multiple types of drugs and performance enhancers? It has always been difficult to draw any straight lines, since Lyle was always on so many different substances at the same time. What perhaps may be the most promising avenue of research is the possible connection between anabolic steroids and underlying personality disorders. After all, many of the football players who were accused of "roid rage" were no angels to begin with. And domestic violence is no stranger in the NFL locker room. Then again, neither were steroids. In Lyle's case, even before he had discovered steroids, he was being physically abused by his father and fighting other kids on the street. He admitted he was violent simply by nature. And then add the years of underreported concussions that may have been exacerbated by or led to Chronic Traumatic Encephalopathy (CTE) of the brain. This steroids-CTE connection is a working theory on why the wrestler Chris Benoit killed himself and his family.

But what actual scientifically published research is out there on anabolic steroids? Here is a little home test you can take. On the left are reported symptoms of anabolic steroid abuse. On the right are two columns, one for strong scientific evidence and one for limited scientific evidence. Go ahead and mark down which symptoms you think have strong evidence and which have limited evidence in the scientific community.

Symptom	Strong Scientific Evidence	Limited Scientific Evidence
Cardiovascular Disease		
Masculinization of Females		
Kidney Failure		
Increased Aggression ("Roid Rage")		
Mania/Depression		
Acne		
Mental and Physical Dependence		
Prostate Cancer		

Now let's see how you did. You will see that everything on that list except for prostate cancer actually has strong scientific evidence to back up its existence.

Symptom	Strong Scientific Evidence	Limited Scientific Evidence
Cardiovascular Disease or Enlarged Heart	X	
Masculinization of Females	X	
Kidney Failure	X	
Increased Aggression ("Roid Rage")	X	
Mania/Depression	X	
Acne	X	
Mental and Physical Dependence	X	
Prostate Cancer		X

So if we know that the connections exist and there is scientific evidence to back it up, what's the dilemma? The controversy arises because some symptoms are more common while others are known, but rare. And like any medication, anabolic steroids can have either rare or common side effects. In doctor-prescribed medications, it's the rare versus common side effects that help decide if a drug makes it to market and if the benefits outweigh the risks. So, let's repeat the exercise now, but see if you can choose those symptoms that are well recognized and those that are more rare.

Symptom	Well Recognized	Rare
Cardiovascular Disease or Enlarged Heart		
Masculinization of Females		
Increased Aggression ("Roid Rage")		
Mania/Depression		
Liver Tumors		
Mental and Physical Dependence		

Let's see how you fared. Below are the completed boxes. You will see that about half the symptoms are well recognized and half are rare. Particularly interesting is the differentiation between mania/depression and increased aggression. Documented increases in mania or depression are actually more often recognized than the stereotypical "roid rage" or hyperaggression.

Symptom	Well Recognized	Rare
Cardiovascular Disease or Enlarged Heart	X	

Masculinization of Females	X	
Kidney Failure		X
Increased Aggression ("Roid Rage")		X
Mania/Depression	X	
Liver Tumors		X
Mental and Physical Dependence	X	

Because of ethical dilemmas, long-term scientific studies on steroid use have not been completed. As a result, users who began in the 1980s and have continued to use them are just now entering their 50s and 60s, and long-term effects like cancer and cardiovascular disease may just now begin to raise their heads. Dr. Charles Yesalis is a well-known steroid expert, motorcycle rider, and gun range enthusiast. He tried three times to get funding for a long-term study, and three times he was denied. After the third strike, he quit trying. So now, he continues to speak out about steroid abuse but admits there is still a behavioral connection that needs to be studied. He defines roid rage as a "spontaneous violent behavior of magnitude that the law becomes involved." Normally, he says, despite a documented increase in aggression from testosterone and anabolic steroids, especially in animal models, social norms in humans are still able to rein in the heightened aggression. He also cautions that connections are hard to make, since, in his research, steroid users are also prone to other drug use.

Behind closed doors, the bodybuilding and sports communities don't seem to care about this lack of research. And in the end, maybe fans don't care, either. Our society continues to value winning and looking good, which are often two benefits of steroids. To the bodybuilding community, Lyle is sometimes described as someone who, in the end, sold out both his community and steroids. They all knew his brain lymphoma wasn't from steroids. If anything, the story should have been about human growth hormone. The HGH side-effect stories of the time in their community weren't limited to Lyle. And if anything, the biggest problems with nonrecreational drug abuse they saw were with diuretics. But, in the end, Lyle's story needed to fit the narrative of the time. John Romano, Lyle's former gym training partner, thinks the audience then and now also needs to be addressed differently. To him, the cheating athlete isn't whom we should be targeting for discussion. We should be targeting the majority of users, i.e., "regular guys who want to look good and fend off the ravages of time."

Regarding as the discussion with athletes, maybe focusing on professionals is the wrong way to go. Everyone knows sports is big business involving larger-than-life athletes doing larger-than-life things. Dr. Yesalis calls it "part of the entertainment package." So, in that sense, Lyle was doing what Lyle was "supposed to" do as an athlete. Where we should be spending our time, he says, is on the high school and junior high school athlete. Professionals know how to cheat the system, but we might actually be able to identify and counsel younger athletes more easily.

Lyle shed a lot of light on the epidemic of steroid abuse, but perhaps making him the face of the dangers was not the right choice given the complexity of the man himself. For many who knew him, it was hard to separate how much of Lyle Alzado was Lyle and how much was the steroids. Which was the greater destructive force eating at him from the inside out? Was it the little boy filled with rage who narrowly survived the "house of horrors," or was it the physical effects of years of performance-enhancing and other drug use? He clearly was a tortured soul, and his life was cut short, not just by his steroid abuse, but also in his quest to find inner validation. Media coverage and the attempt to connect his steroid abuse to his brain lymphoma backfired. To those who used steroids, the media's credibility was lost. The scientific community bristled at any further research. As a result, in his attempt to bring steroids out of the shadows and into the spotlight of the national conversation, Lyle may have inadvertently driven the cobra snake deeper underground.

4

Len Bias and "Biased" Drug Laws

SOMETIMES IN OUR ATTEMPTS TO make things better, we cast too wide a net of change. We can make the mistake of not being specific enough at the beginning of our efforts. When this happens, the cobra snake ensures there is unintended collateral damage with our trawl. Such was the case when the European Union implemented its Common Fisheries Policy, or CFP. Under this law, the EU had hoped to reduce overfishing of certain species. It became illegal to bring on land certain types of fish. Often these fish were over a quota, below a certain size, or part of a species that was not permitted to be sold at all. Since the fishermen's nets would bring in a range of all sorts of species and sizes, this led to a large dumping of fish back into the ocean—fish that likely had already died by the time the ship reached land or those that were either of poor quality or of a species that would not fetch a good price at the market.

This practice came under widespread scrutiny following a campaign started by a TV chef named Hugh Fearnley-Whittingstall. Hugh was the host of a British Channel 4 TV series called River Cottage, which followed the bespectacled Brit and his mop of wavy hair on a quest for food sustainability. After witnessing the large-scale fish discards himself, Hugh was overcome with outrage. He left the successful series in

2010 to focus on setting up and promoting the newly established Fish Fight campaign. According to his group's one-minute documentary, half of the fish caught in the North Sea are thrown back dead as part of discarding practices. His group estimates almost a million tons of fish are wasted every year. The British Michael Moore of food sustainability even took his campaign to Brussels, where he confronted several fisheries and marine officials on camera at the House of Parliament. Buoyed by his efforts, the campaign snagged nearly 900,000 signatures on a petition to end the process of discarding.

Pressured from the media and public outcry, the European Union modified its Common Fisheries Policy, and a ban on discards was enacted. Starting in 2016 and progressing over the following years, a progressive ban on discarding has been implemented. The hope is that by banning discards, fishermen will employ more selective methods in how they fish. If the fish they bring ashore (called "landing") are counted as part of their quota regardless of their market value, then they will hopefully be more selective in what they catch. In essence, the discarding ban is an attempt to override the fishing quotas that led to the discarding in the first place. Under the new rules, the landing quotas will be increased. With these increased landing quotas, the challenge will soon be whether the fishermen discard fish unseen offshore to preserve their landing quotas or bring everything they catch on shore but risk having to use smaller fish with less market value in their allotment. There is a chance that there could become an "oversupply" problem, as well.

Fishing quotas, however, are not wholly evil. In fact, it's been the lack of fishing quotas that has been attributed to EU boats overfishing and decimating fish populations off of North Africa. The sea bass was a traditionally nonquota species, and its population has significantly declined. Discards, too, are not always a bad thing. Many marine animals including birds and mammals have adapted and grown to rely on the waste generated by human activity. In a study published in the journal *Nature Communication*, researchers out of Glasgow actually looked at this concept and concluded that banning discards could also have its own unintended ecological consequences. Instead, the authors argued, we need to focus on being more selective in all aspects of the process, both in fishing and discarding practices.

Another more humorous example of not being selective enough at the beginning of a ban takes us to Scotland, this time about 260 miles from the North Sea, to a steel processing town. Scunthorpe's population is about 82,300 people—the product of the incorporation of five separate villages that all found their way together under the steel industry. Today, there are steam-train rides around the massive steelworks and accompanying railway tracks that have given the town its reputation for approximately 100 years. Scunthopre and steel have become synonymous. However, in 1996, the town gained notoriety for something else.

At the end of the 20th century, the Internet was working its way across the world, connecting countries from all over the globe. One of the biggest platforms was AOL. The residents of the town who tried to sign up for their own accounts soon came across a stumbling block. They were unable to enter the name of their hometown into their profiles. Other residents noticed that the town's name was blocked or banned from websites. One customer was told by AOL customer support that, for sign-in purposes, his hometown was now renamed to Scunthope. Confused, the residents of the UK's steel production center began to look for answers and discovered that AOL's profanity filter had flagged the small town. Scunthorpe had been banned for the four-letter word that governed the majority of its first syllable. Today, the small steel-town's name lives on as a description of when Internet algorithms go wrong and unintentionally block emails, websites, and forum posts due to misunderstood profanity. This "Scunthorpe Effect" is another example of the cobra snake at work and what can go wrong if consequential actions are too broad at their beginning.

WE CAN TRACE THE ORIGIN of a similar effect to the college basketball court.

Mike Krzyzewski is one of the most successful basketball coaches in NCAA history, and as the head coach of Duke University, he and his team have faced off against some of the greatest players in basketball history. Krzyzewski once told the *Washington Post*, "During my years as an ACC coach, the two most dominant players we've faced were Michael Jordan and Len Bias". While Michael Jordan is one of the most recognized names on the planet for basketball, the name of Len Bias has maintained notoriety for over 30 years in the legal war on drugs.

Bias was a star college player for the University of Maryland and was selected as the second overall pick in the 1986 NBA draft by the Boston Celtics, where he would have played alongside such legends as Larry Bird, Robert Parrish, and Kevin McHale. But on June 19, 1986, at 6:30 a.m., a 911 operator received a call from a friend of Len Bias named Brian Tribble:

Dispatcher: "P.G. County Emergency."
Tribble: "Yes, I would like to have an ambulance come to . . . 1103 Washington Hall. It's an emergency. It's Len Bias. He just went to Boston and he needs some assistance."
Dispatcher: "What are you talking about?"
Tribble: "Huh?"
Dispatcher: "What are you talking about?"
Tribble: "I'm talking about someone needs . . . Len Bias needs help."

Just two days after he was drafted in the first round to the NBA at the age of 22, Bias died of cardiac arrhythmia caused by a cocaine overdose. The events that led up to the tragedy are still somewhat in question, but strong efforts have been made to piece together what transpired that fateful night. Police believed that when Bias collapsed, he was in a dorm room on campus where he lived in Washington Hall. Three people were with him about 6:30 a.m. Two of them were his teammates Terry Long and David Gregg. The third was his friend who called 911, but also a suspected drug dealer, Brian Tribble. It was Tribble who was charged with providing the fateful cocaine to Bias.

Two days after the NBA draft, Len had returned home with his father after visiting Reebok to discuss an endorsement deal. Len met with his father, brother, and sister at his parents' home. He gave out new shoes with a smile. He waited around for his mother but decided he wanted to go back up to Maryland to celebrate with his friends. He said good-bye to his father and began the drive back to the university.

He called ahead to his friend Brian, who had a girl over at his apartment. Len arrived, and they dropped the friend off and then headed to Town Hall Liquors. It was there that Len signed an autograph for the cashier. According to Tribble, the two then headed straight to Washington Hall on campus, where Len's friends and teammates were waiting. Len arrived, and he and Tribble met up with Terry Long and David Gregg. It's at this point that Tribble recalls Len saying not to worry, that Terry and David were "cool" with what they did—-meaning they were OK with drugs being used.

Once in Terry Long's room, the four of them began drinking. Soon after, someone supposedly brought out some cocaine, and the group began to pass the drug around on a mirror. A few players would come in and out of room 1103, but each time, the group hid the cocaine out of sight in a drawer until the visitors left. After a few hours, Len remarked he was a little tired and lay back on the bed to close his eyes, still making conversation. Suddenly, Bias went into seizures, his whole body shaking the dorm-room bed. The three other friends, drunk on beer and liquor and high on cocaine, didn't know what to do. Quickly, Tribble had an idea. He would call his mom. His sister had a seizure disorder, so maybe his mom would know what to do for Len. This was a big deal, Len was a big deal, but the last thing they wanted to do was call the police. Then, before they knew it, Len stopped breathing. Now it was a life-or-death matter, so they gave in and Tribble called 911.

Long and Gregg woke up other players, who came into the room and saw Len passed out. Soon, the paramedics arrived and began to work on "Lenny." Keith Gatlin, another Maryland teammate, called Len's parents. His mother answered, unsure of what was going on. After a few minutes of questioning, she informed her husband that

"Frosty," as they called Len, had suffered a seizure and was being brought to the hospital. At first, they were told the wrong hospital, so it took some time before his parents arrived. By the time they arrived, the 22-year-old was already hooked up to a ventilator, as he was unable to breath on his own. It was much later that the family was informed there was nothing more doctors could do. Len Bias had passed away. The city poured its heart out for the Bias family. Jesse Jackson spoke at his funeral. Ronald Reagan sent a card to the family. To have someone on the brink of greatness be tragically and suddenly taken away was a shocking experience. The first flowers to arrive to Len's house were from none other than the man whose legacy Bias was supposed to inherit—Michael Jordan. The second batch came from someone who was supposed to be his Hall of Fame teammate in Boston—Larry Bird. Each set of flowers represented the loss of a dream suddenly not realized.

Not long after his funeral, a new narrative began to surface—a narrative of fame, women, partying, and drugs set along the backdrop of Washington, DC, inner-city streets. To many who knew and were close with Lenny, this was a side of him they never knew. What became even more unclear through investigation was Bias's actual history with drugs. Initially, the autopsy report had said this was his first time using cocaine, but later this was amended to say he could have used drugs before. It was noted that there was damage to his heart muscles, but toxicologists could not connect cocaine to that finding. There were also conflicting reports as to how the cocaine entered his body. One medical examiner suggested that he either sniffed or inhaled the cocaine. Redness in his trachea suggested he may have inhaled, or smoked, the drug. Another report stated the cocaine was found in his stomach as if he had ingested it. The smoking theory was later disputed and the redness attributed to vomiting or placing instruments in his trachea for ventilation. This left either snorting or ingesting. There were even conflicting reports whether alcohol was present in his system when he died. Even the events of the night were in question, with some witnesses saying Len left a college party and then came back later, perhaps with drugs. Police even found a bag of cocaine in his car, but prosecutors alleged that Tribble put it there after Bias collapsed. In a testimony, however, a friend of Len who was a police officer had moved Len's car and searched it for personal belongings after he was pronounced dead. At that time, that particular officer did not see the bag hidden behind the dashboard or the cocaine that had spilled out onto the floor. Other officers later found the bag. Finally, officers found cut straws and a small vial of cocaine crystals as well as beer and a bottle of cognac in the dumpster outside the dorms. Some reports even included a water pipe that could be used to smoke drugs. Of course, another news report said police didn't find anything in the dumpsters outside of the dorm. In other words, no one has a solid understanding of how the events that night actually unfolded or what exactly led to Bias's brain activity being interrupted and subsequent fatal heart attack. The majority of those who were involved or investigating could say that cocaine was likely the culprit in one form or another.

What also piqued the interest of investigators was the level of purity of the cocaine. The purity was of such a high level that it could only have come from someone high up on the drug deal chain. Police pointed their fingers at Brian Tribble, and everyone was brought before a grand jury. Eventually, Tribble turned himself in. Not long after, the University of Maryland athletic department and basketball team fell apart as resignations were forced and players departed. Tribble was found not guilty by a jury. Ironically, investigators later said that while Tribble was a low-level dealer before Bias's death, the tragedy involving Len actually made him a bigger dealer through his infamous association. Tragedy would strike again for the Bias family in 1990, when Len's younger brother was shot while leaving a shopping center after an argument in a jewelry store with a jealous husband of the salesclerk.

Len Bias's death was one of the youngest drug-related deaths in professional sports and received significant media attention during a time when the US government was focusing its message regarding the war on drugs. The death of the young basketball player, however, was just the final linchpin in a political machine that was building up four years earlier, beginning in 1982. In that year, Congress had been focusing its efforts and attention on enacting various bills that concerned themselves with terrorism and pharmaceutical packaging after a scare following the tampering of Tylenol bottles in pharmacies. Drugs were not on the main legislative docket, but as Congress was about to adjourn, Democratic Senator Joe Biden and Republican Chairman of the Senate Judiciary Committee Strom Thurmond included a proposal for a drug czar position.

Biden was a strong advocate for the need of a drug "czar," but he met resistance from the office of the attorney general. At that time, the associate attorney general happened to be future New York City mayor Rudolph Giuliani, who did not support the idea. He described the bill as "naive, simplistic, and hopelessly flawed." The opposition gained traction all the way up to President Ronald Reagan, and despite the bipartisan support of Biden and Thurmond, Reagan sided with the bill's opponents and allowed the bill to fall by the wayside via a "pocket" veto. When the bill fell through, it was felt throughout political circles, and the loss became a public embarrassment to Thurmond. As the Republican committee chairman, Thurmond, people assumed, would have gained the approval of a Republican president following the efforts of a Republican-majority Senate in putting the legislation together and bringing it to the president's desk.

As a result, Thurmond worked diligently on a new bill. Most notably, he found allies in Republican Senator Orrin Hatch and Democratic Senator Ted Kennedy. Then, in 1983, the Comprehensive Crime Control Act was introduced in Congress. It was the first comprehensive revision of the US criminal code since the early 1900s and was a very large bill encompassing many different acts. One of these was the Sentencing Reform Act, which authorized the creation of the United States Sentencing Commission. The purpose of the commission was to create guidelines for the sentencing of federal criminal acts that included tougher sentences for drug dealers.

In September of 1984, a political budget battle was being waged between the Democratic House and Republican Senate. Earlier in the year, President Reagan had accused the Democrats of "dragging their feet" on a crime bill, even as the Republican-led Senate had approved their own version. As the fiscal year was expiring, the Democratic-led House of Representatives faced a government shutdown unless spending measures were approved. When it came time to vote, Republican Dan Lungren from California, a leading anticrime member of Congress, attached the crime reform package to the vote at the last minute. This gave the Democrats only five minutes on the floor to debate the issue that now included crime reform or risk a government freeze. The November elections were only five weeks away, and a government shutdown would have boded poorly for the voting Democrats. Therefore, despite not fully reviewing hundreds of pages of legislation, the Democrats did not want to appear unsupportive of the president's comprehensive crime bill, and many voted to pass the appropriations bill. The Democrats were furious they were manipulated by the Republicans to pass the act, and this became the background of what happened in 1986 following Bias's death.

In 1986, one year after Alzado retired from football and two years after the appropriations bill vote, the Democrats were vying to take back the senate from the Republican Party. At the same time, crack cocaine was suddenly all over the news. Over the summer, *Newsweek* had called crack the biggest story since Vietnam and Watergate. Its June 16th cover carried the title "Crack and Crime." *Time Magazine* labeled it "the issue of the year." The CBS News show *48 Hours* aired a documentary called "48 Hours on Crack Street," which was seen by fifteen million viewers.

And then suddenly, basketball sensation Len Bias was reported dead from a drug overdose. Bias was the second overall draft pick in the NBA and was headed to Boston. When Bias died, the city of Boston was hit emotionally. The Boston Celtics had just rebounded after a heart-breaking loss in the 1985 NBA Championship to Kareem Abdul-Jabbar's Los Angeles Lakers and rose back to become the 1986 NBA Champions. The Celtics won the series on June 8th, the NBA draft occurred on June 17th, and Bias overdosed on June 19th. A few weeks later, Congress returned from its 4th of July break. House Speaker Thomas "Tip" O'Neill was a Democratic leader representing Boston and saw the tragedy as a tipping point for national concern. Prior to his death, Len Bias was already well known in the DC area, having grown up only thirty minutes away in Landover, Maryland, and was poised to become Boston's next great basketball player. O'Neill hoped that the raw emotion of the Bias tragedy would help push forward a bill against drugs that could then help the Democrats reclaim the Senate in the 1986 election. In this way, the Democrats would be seen as being tough on crime when voters looked to the ballots in November. Suddenly, government committees of all kinds in the Senate and House of Representatives were drafting antidrug and anticrime legislation. In the span of a few weeks during the summer of 1986, committees that usually had nothing to do with drugs—such as the committees on agriculture, education, labor, and ways and means—were drafting antidrug and anti-crime legislation. At the time, Congress only had a few weeks between returning in July and breaking again in August, so things were moving at a rapid pace.

Shortly after Labor Day, the House passed its version of the Anti-Drug Abuse Act of 1986. After passing the Senate, the bipartisan bill was signed by President Reagan on October 27, 1986. The bill included further mandatory minimum sentences for drug dealers. It also housed sections for money laundering, prohibition on interstate sales of drug paraphernalia, invoking cooperation of foreign nations in the war on drugs, and drug-free schools and education programs. Further, likely inspired by Tribble's relationship with Bias, the law called for life imprisonment of a person who distributed drugs that resulted in the death of another person (often referred to as the singular "Len Bias Law"). Together, in political and legal circles, these 1986 laws have become collectively known as the "Len Bias Laws."

From 1979 to 1989, Eric Sterling was the assistant counsel to the judiciary committee of the US House of Representatives and had helped write federal laws concerning issues such as firearms, pornography, money laundering, and organized crime. As part of the law, Congress had to decide on which threshold quantity of drugs would be prosecuted under federal law. As a junior staffer, Sterling was considered the "drug expert" for legislative purposes. Much of his efforts at the time were involved with how to deal with "designer" or synthetic drugs as new drugs were being developed. He and his subcommittee comembers were working on how to define the drugs so they could ban not only the currently known drugs, but also those that had not yet been invented. Due process within the law required them to be very specific in the legislation. Additionally, the 1984 Sentencing Commission had not yet taken effect, so it was up to Sterling to come up with guidance on sentencing for high-level drug traffickers.

Sterling initially proposed following the definitions used by the DEA to classify drug traffickers into four classes. The classification was largely based on policies looking at the amounts of drugs seized in places where international drug trafficking took place, such as Miami. It turns out, though, that his number-one informant was a pathological liar who made up his qualifications. When the language was brought forward for markup by the subcommittee, the Democratic congressman from Kentucky Romano Mazzoli objected that the large amounts would not be applicable in towns that are less urban, such as his in Louisville. Sterling understood that drug traffickers did not typically go to these kinds of towns to do major international drug deals and the impetus behind the statute was not that it should be applied in these towns, but rather be applicable to places like Miami, New York, and Houston. Other members, however, agreed with Mazzoli, and as the congressional committee was in such "enormous haste," Sterling quickly came back with newer, smaller thresholds that were adopted without any further hearings a day or two before Congress adjourned for the Labor Day holiday. The resulting trigger threshold became five grams of a mixture or substance containing a *detectable* amount of crack cocaine. Once this threshold was met, it would trigger a minimum sentence of five years if convicted of a drug-related crime. In contrast, the threshold for a mixture or substance containing a *detectable* amount of *powder* cocaine became 500 grams.

Following the 1986 law, the simple possession of a controlled substance without the intent to distribute was only a misdemeanor. As a result, there was a potential loophole that someone could possess a controlled substance but not intend to distribute it. But in 1988, as the congressional "War on Drugs" continued, a new drug law aimed at closing this loophole. A new bill was introduced making crack cocaine the only drug with a mandatory minimum penalty for a first offense of simple possession. With the Anti-Drug Act of 1988 (also an election-year cycle), it deemed the simple possession of five grams of crack cocaine (even without any evidence of an intent to distribute) would also carry a minimum of five years, up to 20 years. On the other hand, there was no quantity of the powder-form cocaine (in the absence of documented evidence of an intent to distribute) that, if simply possessed, would automatically trigger a greater sentence. As a result of this vagueness, the courts later ruled that possession of a "quantity" could be so substantial that it could be inferred that there was an intent to distribute. Often, "expert witnesses" from the police narcotics squad or DEA would testify that in their expert opinion, among other circumstantial evidence, quantity X was too large to be possessed for the exclusive use by the defendant and that an intent to distribute could be inferred.

Under the 1986 mandatory minimum sentencing laws (the collective "Len Bias Laws"), 500 grams of powder cocaine carried the same sentence as five grams of crack cocaine, despite the fact that five grams of powdered cocaine contained 100 times the amount of crack cocaine. This 100:1 bias toward crack cocaine possession was based on the public perception that the crack form of the drug had a higher link to crime and a greater propensity for causing an epidemic of "crack babies" to be born. These myths have since been proven false. Studies have shown that similar biological effects are found in developing brains that are exposed to either crack or powdered cocaine. The violence related to the crack drug trade has been shown to be similar to crimes associated with the illegal trafficking and sale of other drugs and not necessarily specific to crack itself.

What has been proven is that the crack form of the drug tends to be cheaper and therefore more widely used by African American drug abusers, while the powder form is often more expensive and therefore tends to be more accessible to more affluent and/or Caucasian drug abusers. Data compiled by the United States Sentencing Commission in 2006 illustrated that African Americans are more likely to be convicted of crack cocaine offenses, while whites are more likely to be convicted of powder cocaine offenses. Ironically, while many in the media had assumed that Bias—an African American—had died of a crack overdose, he actually died of an overdose of powdered cocaine.

Data have also shown that the overall problem is further compounded in that white drug abusers are less likely to be prosecuted for drug offenses, and when they are prosecuted, they are more likely to be acquitted. Furthermore, if they are convicted, they are much less likely to be sent to prison. Since the Len Bias laws took effect, racial differences in drug-related sentencing have become even more apparent. Before the 1986 act, the average federal drug sentence for African Americans was 11 percent higher than for whites. Four years later, after the act was initiated, the average federal drug sentence for African Americans was 49 percent higher. Also since 1986, there has been a disproportionate impact on African American women. Incarceration rates for all African Americans since 1986 have largely been driven by drug convictions, and data have shown an increase of 800 percent since 1986. This is compared to an increase of 400 percent for women of all races for the same time period.

Another problem with the law was that it was initially intended to take down large-scale drug dealers as part of the 1980s "War on Drugs." Yet, when used in practice, the law largely focuses on lower-level dealers due to the trigger levels. Here is an illustrative scenario from a legal journal article in 2003: A high-level supplier can sell 450 grams of powder cocaine down the chain until just a small quantity reaches several street dealers. If one of those street dealers takes that much smaller amount and cooks it with baking soda to produce a 5.1-gram rock of crack and gets caught selling it, he or she will face a mandatory minimum sentence of five years. If the higher-level drug supplier who had the 450 grams of powder cocaine had been caught earlier, he or she would have less than the 500-gram trigger for powder cocaine and therefore would not face the same mandatory minimum sentence as the low-level street dealer at the end of the supply chain.

In 2010, through the bipartisan Fair Sentencing Act under President Obama, the crack amount trigger was significantly changed to 28 grams, or 1 ounce, largely due to a demonstrable disparate weight on sentencing crack over powder cocaine. As a result, the composition trigger imbalance of 100:1 toward crack was reduced to 18:1. Data from the time showed that it was the street-level dealers and not high-level drug traffickers who were subject to the mandatory minimum penalty at the highest rate. A more recent report in 2017 has shown a general downward trend in the percentage of offenders convicted of a drug offense carrying a mandatory minimum penalty. The largest decrease was for the street-level dealer, down from about 61 percent in 2009 to about 32 percent in 2016. Yet, although the mandatory drug sentences were aimed at "serious" and "major" traffickers with initial intent of the 1980s drug laws, the data indicate that mandatory minimum penalties have been and are still applied much more broadly. In fact, in 2016, over half (52.8 percent) of drug offenders convicted of an offense that carried a drug mandatory minimum penalty faced mandatory minimum penalties of 10 years or more. And among the total number of drug offenders in federal prison, almost three-quarters (72.3 percent) were convicted of an offense carrying a mandatory minimum penalty. Now, more recently at the end of 2018, a significant bipartisan act of legislation aimed at reforming the Len Bias-era disproportionate sentencing laws was signed into law. The so-called FIRST STEP Act allows the 2010 Fair Sentencing Act to be applied retroactively, affecting approximately 200,000 people in federal prisons.

Proponents of drug law reform such as Sterling, however, don't feel the needle has moved enough. In fact, it may even be on the wrong gauge. Since he left the government in 1989, Sterling has been the executive director of The Criminal Justice Policy Foundation, a private nonprofit organization that "helps educate the nation about criminal justice issues and failed global drug policy." He feels that there has been "an enormous injustice" because of the harsh sentences implied by the Len Bias laws. During Obama administration budget battles, there was a significant decrease in spending support for prosecution of drug offenders. So, while there are trends toward fewer federal drug cases and fewer federal drug prisoners, this may have been just due to less overall drug prosecution. For Sterling, the "underlying problem" is not that there are "fewer unjust sentences," but a failure to allocate proper punishment for drug offenders. In fact, most of the drug reform laws focused on crack offenders but failed to address most of the other drugs we see in society today.

Since helping to draft the Len Bias laws, Sterling feels that over-zealous prosecution of drug offenders actually worsens the problem. To him, this method of prosecution increases crime, allows drug dealers to rise to greater limits of power, and stigmatizes drug users as criminals, which in turn inhibits their abilities to seek adequate treatment for their drug addictions. As a result, these drug abusers become at increased risk for overdose—the very thing that killed Len Bias.

Having followed drug policy for over 30 years, Sterling has accepted that the tragedy of Len Bias was exploited for political reasons: "We engaged in an experiment and learned tragically that it didn't work and we need to move in a new direction. We need to help those with drug problems manage their disorder and reduce the issues of drug abuse from being the most important aspect of their lives to the least important aspect." In today's society, it is easier for people to connect on social media and in other ways follow tragic events, especially those involving celebrities. Yet, for someone like Sterling who has been part of congressional legislative committees, public outcry may not be enough. What happened in 1986 he largely attributes to leaders in Congress needing a rallying cry during an election cycle coupled with misinformation from a NARC source who proved to be untruthful. Sterling uses this analogy to sum up the exploitation of Len Bias's 1986 death, "In real estate they say the most important rule is 'location, location, location.' Maybe the most famous rule in politics is 'it's all about the timing.'"

So with Len Bias's death, the tragic loss of a young African American star athlete to cocaine led to a poorly managed drug war on crack and a broken criminal justice system for millions of other young African Americans that we are still continuing to legislatively reform over 30 years later. Like the fishing trawls in the North Sea, perhaps not being selective enough up front led to an unexpectedly high catch yield and subsequent mass discards. Had the Len Bias laws been more properly focused, the war on drugs may have been fought much differently, and the criminal justice system and those affected by it might be standing in a different place today.

5

Hank Gathers, Dale Lloyd, and Athlete Screening

IT WAS TO BE ONE of the most important medical drugs of our generation. It was to be the biggest-selling pharmaceutical in history. It was going to save lives. Phase III trials were well underway involving over 15,000 patients across 260 centers in seven countries. Pfizer research chief John LaMattina told analysts, "We believe this is the most important new development in cardiovascular medicine in years." Then, just two days later, it all came crashing down.

It was 7 a.m. on December 2, 2006, when the phone rang at LaMattina's Connecticut home. It was early on a Saturday, and he was in the shower. *Who would be calling at this time?* he wondered to himself. He sensed something was wrong. Maybe it was one of his children. Still wet from the shower, he walked over to his office and answered the phone. What he heard made him sit down. Their new wonder drug was killing more people than it was helping. The trial had to be shut down.

The drug trial involved two arms. One-half of patients would take Pfizer's well-known cholesterol drug, Lipitor. The other half would also take Lipitor but would add their new darling, torcetrapib. During the trial, on the first day of each month, independent monitors would present data on the progress of the drug trial. Only they, and not

Pfizer, were privy to these results. This time, however, the data were too overwhelming. Eighty-two patients in the experimental group had died, compared to 51 patients in the control group. Not only was this number higher, but it was *statistically* higher, meaning in this case that the odds this was due to random chance were less than 99 out of 100 (statisticians refer to this as a p-value less than 0.01).

The impetus behind the trial was doctors' and scientists' thought processes on reducing cardiovascular disease by altering the levels of "good" versus "bad" cholesterol—a model, as it turned out, that was unfortunately too simplified. Medical students and doctors in training had long been taught that there were two types of cholesterol in the body. LDLs, or "low-density lipoproteins," are fat molecules that help transport fatty cholesterol to the body's cells, where it becomes a building block for other things. But if too many LDL molecules clogged up the highways of the circulatory system, then plaques could form in the arteries. If these plaque buildups ruptured, they could set off a cascade that resulted in blood clots blocking an artery. This in turn could lead to a devastating stroke or deadly heart attack. HDLs, or "high-density lipoproteins," were considered the good guys. They swept through the blood and helped clean up excess cholesterol and bring it back to where it belonged, in the liver. So, scientists and doctors thought, in a manner of oversimplification, if we lower "bad" LDL levels, and raise "good" HDL levels, then we can start to win the fight against heart disease.

In the 1980s, researchers began to focus on a family of drugs called "statins" that could reduce cholesterol levels, specifically LDL levels. It wasn't until the 2000s that HDL-raising drugs were really introduced. In 1999, Pfizer first gave patients torcetrapib and, buoyed by Phase I trials, the company embarked on Phase II trials in 2000. A small clinical trial of 19 patients published in the *New England Journal of Medicine* in 2004 showed promise in raising HDL levels. The way the drug worked was by inhibiting a protein called CETP that converted HDL to LDL. Scientists were first alerted to the importance of CETP when they noticed that patients with decreased CETP activity due to mutations seemed to have elevated HDL levels. Phase III trials began in 2003, and the only blip seemed to be a small increase in patients' blood pressures.

By 2004, Pfizer had launched its new trial comparing use of its widely used cholesterol-lowering drug Lipitor plus a placebo pill to the use of Lipitor with the even-better torcetrapib. By the end of 2006, following the findings of the independent trial monitors, the drug was abandoned completely, and Pfizer's $800 million investment would go down the tubes. It seemed that simply trying to raise HDL was not the answer, and in fact, the drug being used to accomplish the task appeared to have deadly side-effects. Even the whole "good" vs "bad" model of cholesterol was called into question. Maybe there was another explanation for how cholesterol led to cardiovascular disease events than just the ratio of LDL vs HDL. Maybe it had to do with something else, like inflammation. Studies have even shown that if HDL, a.k.a. the "good" cholesterol, is too high, it can lead to premature mortality in men and women.

The Cobra Effect of the torcetrapib trial shows how when we are given data, especially in complex systems such as the human body, we can't always make accurate predictions with those data. We know there is a problem, and we see a potential solution. But when we try to act on the problem with the data we have, we may not be seeing the whole picture. The data may not apply to all populations. Our model may be flawed. It's deciding which information we actually know and how to best act on that information that can let the cobra snake slip in if we aren't careful.

"GASOLINE ON FIRE." THAT'S HOW Bryant Gumbel described Loyola Marymount University's (LMU) basketball style in 1990. Al Roker had just tossed the segment over to Gumbel, who was sitting at the anchor desk on the *Today Show*. LMU was averaging almost 123 points a game, setting an NCAA record that still stands today. His guests that day were the two stars of the team, Hank Gathers and Bo Kimble. Each dressed up for the appearance, Gathers clad in a black short sleeve silk shirt and Kimble in a gray blazer. Shiny necklaces glittered across their chests. Kimble sported a tight crew cut and Gathers a 1990s flat-top.

A pencil-thin mustache danced atop Gathers's lips as he flashed a big smile. Gumbel had asked Gathers if he thought his 6'7" height would be a challenge to overcome once he played in the NBA. Hank, the self-declared strongest man in the world, swatted the comment away like a defender blocking a jumpshot. "That doesn't bother me," Gathers replied, "because I have the heart the size of a lion." He quickly followed up with "Any lion," as if to say his heart was stronger than any of the other players Gumbel might have been thinking of. Hank might face bigger or more intimidating players, but he would never back down. In fact, he even went toe-to-toe with the NCAA's big man of the era, Shaquille O'Neal. In a game versus Shaq's LSU team, the 7-foot-tall center blocked Gathers's shot 10 or 12 times, but Gathers kept coming back. Not only did he keep coming back, but he would do so right at the big man. It would only be a matter of weeks before we would learn just how important that lion's heart was to Gathers's legacy.

Hank and Bo Kimble had known each other since high school. They had grown up in the Philadelphia projects, and like many inner-city kids, basketball was their ticket out. At first, they found themselves at odds as rivals, but over time their relationship grew much closer as their lives intertwined. Hank had his whole life planned. He would play for a big basketball school, make money as an NBA player, especially as a lottery draft pick, and then retire to do sports broadcasting. On the surface, he was a happy-go-lucky guy, but his real self would be compared by his college coach to Shakespeare's Falstaff, a comical knight who, upon close examination, reveals much depth in character. Hank's particular depth was his heart—his determination to excel and always be better than before. He spent an uneventful year as a freshman, passing the time at USC, before his never-quit attitude found the perfect forge for stoking in the coaching style of Paul Westhead, Loyola Marymount's newest basketball coach.

Westhead had coached the Los Angeles Lakers to an NBA

championship in 1980 by employing what he called "The System." In the system, players take an incredible number of shots, with the theory being that the more shots you take, the more you can make. But the strategy didn't just stop with the math. Players were expected to shoot the ball every 8 seconds or less. Each player would sprint as hard as he could to a designated spot at the far end of the basketball court. By running as fast as they could from the beginning tip-off to the final buzzer, they knew they would eventually break the other team, both physically and mentally. To the uninitiated, it looked like basketball without a strategy. But for kids coming from a life of streetball in the projects of Philly, it was perfect. For three years straight, the LMU team would lead the nation in scoring per game, averaging around 120 points each game. Mental and physical toughness was of the utmost importance. The players would become conditioned like Navy Seals. Training would regularly include sprinting up a sand dune whose top was barely visible from the bottom. And the whole time, Gathers loved it. He got stronger and faster and quickly became one of the NCAA's top scorers and top rebounders. He was only the second player in history to lead the nation in both scoring and rebounding. And it was the rebounding that Hank was the most proud of. It was a way to separate himself from the crowd of other NBA prospects who all were breathing the same rarefied air. He called it his "bread and butter." It was what the scouts would notice. And most important, he said, rebounding comes from the heart.

On December 9, 1989, The Hank and Bo show, as LMU's high-scoring system was called, was in full effect. The duo was leading their team against UC Santa Barbara. With about fourteen minutes left in the game, Gathers drove to the basket and was fouled, sending him to the free-throw line. Gathers, a right-handed shooter, was getting ready to shoot the free throws left-handed, as he had done all season. You see, for Gathers, a basketball Greek hero, free throws were his Achilles' heel. He just couldn't make them. As a result, in his last college season, he tried switching to his nondominant hand for free throws.

The crowd watched as the LMU senior got ready to shoot the first of two free-throws. Suddenly, he began to feel a warm sensation in his feet. The sensation then began to travel up his legs all the way to his head. Feeling something was off, Gathers let the shot fly quickly, missing the basket. Then, before he could brace himself, he suddenly collapsed to the gym floor. At first, his teammates thought the consummate performer was joking. Gathers was lying on his left shoulder, almost as if taking a nap. But it didn't take long to realize something was amiss. A few seconds later, his eyes snapped open and he got up. He walked off the court, holding his hands up like a heavyweight prizefighter. The lion was still proud. The court was still his kingdom. Many people just dismissed it as a freak accident. A fainting spell that was the result of the hot temperature in the gym coupled with the frenetic pace of "The System."

Back in the locker room area, next to the athletic trainer's office, a doctor examined Hank and felt something that drew his concern. Normally, each steady beat of the heart results in a pressure wave within the arteries giving rise to a regular pulse. But Gathers's pulse seemed irregular, which meant the blood was being pumped out of his heart at an irregular rate. If that were happening, it was possible the electrical conducting system of his heart might be experiencing a small malfunction. The doctor decided he needed to send Gathers for some testing: routine cardiac function tests including an electrocardiogram to assess electrical conduction in the heart, and blood tests to rule out a myocardial infarction, or, in other words, a heart attack. It was as if someone suddenly pulled the carpet out from under Gathers. It was like he had just fallen to the floor again. He began to sob. Hank turned to a friend who had just walked in. "I just blew my NBA career," he said.

Hank would undergo a few days of testing, first at Centinela Hospital, where he would be seen by a well-known sports medicine internist in the area; and then later at Daniel Freeman Memorial Hospital in Inglewood, where he would be seen by both cardiologist Dr. Vernon Hattori and electrophysiologist Dr. Charles Swerdlow. The tests were varied, including a treadmill stress test and an electrophysiology test, which involved a catheterization of his blood vessels.

Gathers, who was awake during the catheterization procedure, was extremely upset. All he could think about was getting back on the court, and now this diagnosis and these doctors were keeping him from his future. He was so angry, he refused to see his mother after the testing was done.

After all the tests were completed, the doctors analyzed the results. What they saw was evidence that, for the world's strongest college basketball player and future NBA star, exercise could induce a potentially fatal heart rhythm (an "arrhythmia"). Gathers was informed he had an "enlarged heart." The medical term was hypertrophic cardiomyopathy, meaning the muscles of the heart were bigger than expected and weren't functioning properly. Gathers would need to take a beta-blocker, a medicine that acted on receptors to slow the heart rate down. This would help the heart to fully fill with blood between beats. He would need to take this medicine with meals three times a day and undergo a biopsy of his heart once the season was over. He was also to be tested weekly for proper medication levels. Gathers also promised that, if he felt that same odd body sensation again, he would take himself out of the game. However, so as not to arouse suspicion by the NBA scouts or media, he said his plan would be to fake a stomachache or muscle pull.

LMU's athletic trainer was given a defibrillator to shock Gathers's heart back into line, but its purpose was often kept secret, even from other players, who thought it was actually a Nintendo in his luggage. Hank also hid the fact that for a while, he was wearing a heart monitor during practice. There was some suggestion by those around Hank who knew of his heart issue that he should cash in on a million-dollar insurance policy he had taken out earlier in his college career. This idea seemed to miss the rim, so to speak, to which Hank would grab the rebound and quickly redirect the conversation like a guard throwing a pass downcourt.

Gathers would eventually be cleared to play, but he found that the medicine, Inderal, made him sluggish. He couldn't play at the top of his game. This became especially evident when he returned to his hometown for a game against Philadelphia's Saint Joseph's University. In front of his family and young son, Aaron, he failed to score more than one point in the first half and only 11 points total. This was entirely uncharacteristic for one of the nation's top scorers. Without Gathers's offense, his team struggled. It looked like they were about to lose the game. Fortunately, the other Philadelphian and Gathers's former Dobbins Tech High School teammate, Bo Kimble, would sink a last-second shot to seal the victory for LMU.

It was around this time that Gathers requested that his medication dosage be lowered. It was affecting his game too much. He continued to keep his diagnosis a closely guarded secret, even from many of those close to him, including his child's mother. He also began to miss follow-up testing visits. Dr. Hattori, the cardiologist taking care of him, would call Hank asking where he was, and each time Gathers would tell him he would show up the next day. Predictably, each time, he didn't. Finally, Hattori called Gathers and told him not only that he needed to see him, but also that he wasn't taking enough of the medication to be effective. Unless he increased his dosage, he could not play in the upcoming West Coast Conference tournament games. In what had become somewhat typical, Gathers bristled and protested against the decision. Hattori reminded Hank that at the minimum, he needed to listen to his heart. If it started racing again, he needed to get off the court immediately and call him. In the second game of the regional tournament, Gathers was flying high once again. Six-and-a-half minutes into the game, he caught an alley-oop and slammed the ball into the basket with both hands. The crowd roared. Hank "The Bank" Gathers trotted toward midcourt. And then suddenly, he collapsed again. He tried to get up again. But this time, he didn't. Hank Gathers stayed down.

The team's trainer arrived at his side first, followed by Gathers's aunt and then the two Loyola team doctors. Soon, they were joined by his mother, friend, and brother. His aunt pleaded for someone to do something. They felt he had a pulse, so they held off on the defibrillator. Three minutes later, 911 was called. As they were waiting for the paramedics, they loaded Hank onto a stretcher and brought him outside the gym door into a less public area. At this point, the defibrillator was hooked up and, sensing no pulse, recommended a shock. A total of three shocks were given. Hank briefly lifted his head and opened his eyes. He took two deep breaths, and then his head fell back again. Four minutes after the 911 call, the paramedics arrived and continued CPR on Hank. He was brought to the local hospital, where the ER team continued to work on him. The hospital switchboard lit up, and the crowd outside the ER grew. After one hour, two doctors emerged from the treatment area and walked over to his mother and aunt. Wails of anguish rose from the waiting area. Hank Gathers was no longer alive. The high-flying strongest man in the world had forever been grounded. The heart of a lion no longer beat.

A dark cloud of mourning fell over Loyola Marymount University. Their star player, the charismatic joker, the future NBA superstar, had suddenly died in front of their eyes. Nobody knew what to do next, but as fate would have it, his team had advanced to the NCAA basketball tournament. A discussion was had as to whether to withdraw, but knowing Hank's never-say-die attitude, the team chose to play in Hank's honor. Buoyed by their love for their teammate, they went on a storybook run, defeating several high-ranking teams in the process before losing in the Elite Eight round. In what was perhaps one of the greatest heartfelt moments in sports history, Bo Kimble, in a tribute to his longtime friend and teammate, took his first free throw of the tournament left-handed. The crowd roared its approval.

Gathers's legacy, however, did not end there. Grief-stricken, and in what is often normal human behavior following a tragedy, the family looked around for a reason and someone to blame. Under the direction of lawyers, they began to sue the school and the doctors who treated him. Aaron Crump, his son, would be awarded almost 1.5 million dollars, and the Gathers story would become a textbook medicolegal case to be taught for decades later.

One year later, in 1991, another high-profile basketball player for the Boston Celtics, Reggie Lewis, would also die on the court from a heart-related problem (the role of drugs in this case has been debated). Then, in 1993, Gathers's own cousin would also die on the court at the young age of 17. With so many on-court deaths, the debate on how to prevent these tragedies would grow over the next several years. Calls would be made by many in the medical community to screen college athletes, especially basketball players, with electrocardiograms (EKGs). The EKG could help detect cardiac electrical abnormalities, especially in young black basketball players. The only problem was, nobody could tell how useful these tests would be on a large scale. In fact, it was still unclear how many NCAA college basketball players were at risk for sudden cardiac death. And of that group, how many would be detectable by EKG. Like in many areas of medicine, well-meaning doctors who want to make sure we are doing the right things for patients would find evidence on both sides of the debate, and the results would not be black-and-white.

In 2015, a study was published in *Circulation*, the official medical journal of the American Heart Association. The authors of the study looked back at all levels of NCAA records from 2003 to 2013 and found that during that decade, the rate of sudden cardiac death in Division I male college basketball players was 1 in 5,200 per year. Black male athletes were almost at a 3x higher risk than white male athletes (1 in 15,829 athletes vs. 1 in 45,514). These data prompted the chief medical physician of the NCAA to mandate EKG screening of athletes in an attempt to avoid another Hank Gathers-type situation. This was met by resistance from many team physicians. For one thing, Hank Gathers may have died after not taking his medication. Second, we don't necessarily know the true risk numbers. Third, this may open up schools who don't test up to legal implications. Should an athlete die from a heart irregularity, a school could be held liable if it failed to perform the mandated EKG screening. And fourth, and this is their biggest point, the level of false positives would just be so high that it wouldn't be worth dealing with all the financial and emotional headache of false positives given the infrequent nature of the actual cardiac event. And if a player did have a positive test, what is the implication for denying them a chance to play? And what say does the athlete have in all this?

In general, simply screening for heart problems by a history and physical exam will only catch about 10 percent of the problems in athletes. Many top sports organizations have turned to EKGs for mandatory screening. Supporters of EKG screening will point to studies that say it can detect 90 percent to 95 percent of hypertrophic cardiomyopathy (which is what Gathers died from). That seems like a pretty good screening tool. It can also detect other electrical abnormalities of the heart. But even if a young athlete gets an EKG screen, it may not be read properly. While many doctors are skilled at EKG interpretation, there is a particular niche in reading EKGs of athletes' hearts, since they may not be the same as those of the general population. Defining abnormal EKGs can be a challenge, and as a result, studies have suggested false positive rates ranging from 5 percent all the way up to 20 percent. A 2014 article in the American Heart Association journal *Circulation* put this into perspective: "If ECGs with false-positive results could be reduced to only 5% in the course of screening 10 million individuals (the estimated number of US competitive athletes), screening ECGs would nevertheless identify a formidable obstacle of 500,000 people who required further testing." If you use that same analogy and consider 500,000 NCAA athletes (494,992 students competed in NCAA championship sports in the 2017–18 academic year), 5 percent of that group is 25,000 athletes with false positives that would need to be screened to play college sports.

Therein lies the debate. Is it cost-effective to screen so many athletes? One way to combat the cost of the EKG (estimated at $25 per athlete) is to make sure you are using it in a high-risk population. As the incidence of a particular disease goes up in a specific population, the likelihood of finding a true positive condition will go up and thereby improve cost-effectiveness of the screening tool. In general, the highest-risk populations seem to be male basketball players, football players, and soccer players.

Interestingly, in the same study of the NCAA records from 2003–2013, the most common findings at autopsy of those diagnosed with sudden cardiac death was that nothing was found. In 16 patients, or 25 percent of the athletes studied, there was no definitive evidence of changes in the heart muscles as the cause of death. Only 5 athletes, or 8 percent of the study group, had autopsy-definitive evidence of hypertrophic cardiomyopathy. This is what makes studies of this nature so difficult: it is very hard to definitively say what was the cause of death for many of these athletes. In general, most basketball players will have larger-than-normal hearts. The average size of an NBA basketball player is about 6'7" and 225 pounds. That is clearly not the same size as the average person. On top of that, the heart, like any other muscle, can get bigger with exercise. A 2015 study published by Columbia University, one of the NBA's heart-monitoring institutions, looked at this very issue. Using an echocardiogram, or ultrasound, study of the heart, the doctors found that the average heart of an NBA player was 10 percent larger than the average person's. This was considered normal for this group of athletic giants. Furthermore, African American professional basketball players had hearts even larger than their white counterparts.

Let's look, for example, at a young black male from Philadelphia like Hank Gathers who grew up in the projects. Basketball is one of his few avenues out of the poverty-stricken neighborhood. If he were to stay behind in Philadelphia, the chance of his dying from a gun-related homicide, according to a 2018 study published in the *Annals of Internal Medicine*, would be almost 43 out of every 100,000 men each year. That's 0.043% per year. The chance of sudden cardiac death in NCAA male athletes? That would be .0063% per year. Therefore, is it worth denying this young man the chance to play basketball and potentially improve his life if his chance of dying from gun violence in Pennsylvania is 7x higher than dying suddenly on the basketball court?

And what does the athlete get to decide in all of this? In a more recent example of athlete autonomy debate, we can turn to the neon lights of Miami. After being the starting power forward for the Miami

Heat's 2012 and 2013 back-to-back NBA championships, Chris Bosh was set to take the mantle as leader of the Miami Heat. That crown was previously held by LeBron James, who left Miami to return to his former team, the Cleveland Cavaliers. Bosh had just signed a five-year, $118 million contract, and his future looked bright. The season began, and suddenly Bosh began to feel his breath was short. He even had shooting chest pains. But this was the year to be the big man, so he didn't pay much attention to it and ignored the discomfort. Nevertheless, it kept coming back. Finally, he told the team doctors, and he was quickly sent to the hospital for tests that revealed he had blood clots in his lungs, something called pulmonary embolism. He would miss the rest of the season after undergoing a procedure to remove the clots, but after taking medication to prevent further clots, he returned the next season to the NBA hardwood.

Then in 2016, as he was heading into the All-Star Break, Bosh felt a sharp pain in his calf. The team told the media it was a calf strain, but tests showed a new blood clot in his leg, a distal vein thrombosis (DVT). Doctors quickly cautioned him that a piece of the clot could break off and travel through his blood vessels to his lungs and lead to a sudden death. This was not what Bosh wanted to hear. He became at odds with the doctors and team organization. He wanted to play, but they wouldn't let him.

Chris wouldn't be the first, or the last, athlete to try and ignore a doctor's advice. One of the most notable instances might have been in the case of football lightning rod Terrell Owens's decision to play in Super Bowl XXXIX. Seven weeks before 2005's big game, "T.O." was hit by Roy Williams and suffered a twisting injury that fractured his fibula below the knee but, more important, tore the ligament that connects the two leg bones (the "shinbone" or tibia and the adjacent fibula). He required surgery to stabilize the two bones until the ligament could heal. His surgeon advised him not to play to allow the ligament adequate time to heal, but the Philadelphia Eagles wide receiver played anyways. Much to the surprise of many, Owens had an MVP-like performance with nine catches for 122 yards against the Patriots.

The Eagles would lose the game, but T.O.'s performance was one to remember. He succeeded temporarily despite ignoring doctors' advice, but in his case, the downside of playing was possibly cutting his career short, not his life.

Naturally, Bo Kimble had some advice for NBA star Chris Bosh at the time he was considering coming back: "There are so many other things he could do with his life. Hank Gathers had the same thing, Hank could have been a comedian, an actor or did speaking engagements." Kimble continued, "It's not worth the risk . . . if Hank had the ability to do it again he wouldn't have paid the ultimate price." Fortunately, Bosh would heed his advice and retire from professional basketball. Still, screening controversies in sports haven't stopped with the heart.

On September 24, 2006, Dale Lloyd II wiped the sweat from his brow during what was supposed to be a light Sunday workout on the Rice University football field. The freshman cornerback could tell his teammates were noticing him lagging behind on sprints, something that was uncharacteristic for him. The supplement drink the team trainers gave him earlier mixed with creatine certainly wasn't keeping the coaches off his back. The 19-year-old was breathing heavier than normal, and his legs felt like they were tightening up. He tried to pull himself together for yet another 100-yard sprint. How many had it been? *Sixteen?* he wondered to himself. He tried to shake it off. And then, suddenly, as if someone turned out the lights, everything went black. Dale passed out on the field.

Unexpectedly, just a day later, Dale died. His death was a result of complications related to a genetic condition known as sickle cell trait. Sickle cell trait is when a person inherits only one copy of the sickle cell gene (as opposed to the full two copies—one from each parent). Therefore, most of the time, their red blood cells usually have a normal round appearance. But when the oxygen level in their blood drops, from sprinting for example, the red blood cells change into a more elongated sickle shape and can clog blood vessels. While most people have likely heard of sickle cell disease, many may be unaware that just having the trait can lead to significant and deadly complications. Like sickle cell disease, the sickle cell trait is especially predominant in African American populations. About 1 out of every 12 African Americans has the sickle cell trait. Considering the average college basketball team has 12 players and consists primarily of African American men, that means nearly one player on each NCAA basketball team will have the trait. In 2006, when Dale died, only about 20 percent of universities were testing their athletes for the trait. It certainly wasn't mandatory, and Rice University was in the vast majority of those institutions that didn't routinely screen their players. Following Dale's death, his parents learned about the lack of testing. They found it unacceptable that other parents could lose their child to this condition, and as part of their lawsuit that included the university, the NCAA, and the supplement makers, they pressed for mandatory screening across collegiate sports. As part of the settlement following the Lloyd Family lawsuit, the NCAA began to test routinely for the sickle cell trait. It started with Division I athletes in 2010, DII athletes in 2012, and DIII athletes in 2013.

Soon after the testing began, which athletes could actually opt out of by simply signing a waiver, calls of foul began to rise. In a study from 1982 to 2008, there were 108 nontraumatic deaths across college sports. Deaths related to sickle cell disease were less than 10 percent, while deaths linked to heart problems was significantly higher at 65 percent. One group that was particularly vocal in its disapproval was the American Society of Hematology, accusing the NCAA of overstepping its bounds and acting as reactionary hematologists.

With the support of multiple other medical groups, the society of blood specialists produced a consensus statement rebuking the NCAA and suggesting it focus its efforts on a more effective approach. They felt that there was not necessarily a documented cause and effect of sickle cell trait with exercise-associated deaths. There was an established correlation, but not necessarily causation. They also argued that there is no need to worry about sudden death from overexertion during certain sports such as bowling or golf. Instead, they suggested the NCAA take a page out of the US Army's manual. In a 1987 study, the Army was faced with a 37-fold increased risk of basic training deaths in recruits who carried the sickle cell trait. In response to these data, the Army did not implement routine screening but instead focused on adequate hydration and rest. This in turn, helped to protect the recruits from the dangers of overexertion and hyperthermia. If the NCAA would change their tactic to prevention rather than screening, it could help avoid the legal and ethical pitfalls of denying an athlete a scholarship due to the results of a genetic test or even the likely connection to racial discrimination, since the trait is significantly higher in black athletes.

Twenty-five years later, we still don't know the best way to prevent another tragedy on the basketball court from sudden cardiac death. We don't know if EKG testing is cost-effective for nonprofessional athletes. And what about genetic testing? How deep do we want to dig for answers to prevent a sudden death? What Pandora's box of genetic screening might we open? Is there a gene for jumping higher or more triple-doubles? Should coaches and colleges even be discussing a person's genetic code? Would we base NBA draft order or college scholarships on genetic analysis? Here we are faced with another possible Cobra Effect. When presented with data, how we interpret them and act on them can have long-standing unintended consequences.

6
Ayrton Senna, Dale Earnhardt, and NASCAR's Car of Tomorrow

"ONLY YOU CAN PREVENT FOREST fires" is perhaps the most memorable slogan ever to be uttered by a talking *noncartoon* bear—Smokey Bear, to be precise. Most people know the furry forest ranger as "Smokey" The Bear, but in actuality, his given name was simply Smokey Bear. He first appeared in 1944, two years after Disney's *Bambi* laid bare the devastating effects of forest fires on animal habitats. Hot on the trail of Bambi, other animals began to appear in posters and ad campaigns as part of the National Park System's efforts to curtail forest fires. Unable to employ the young fawn for more than a year, the government organization turned to *New Yorker* art critic and part-time ad man Harold Rosenberg. He first breathed life into the large, friendly bear. Shortly after his creation, he was named Smokey after Smokey Joe Martin, a firefighter who was blinded and burned during a fire rescue. Smokey was further personified when a small black bear cub was actually rescued from a forest fire and sent to live in Washington, DC's national zoo. This cute and cuddly cub provided even more ammunition in the forest service's efforts to combat forest fires at all costs. This effort, however, had its own unintended consequences.

In the early 20th century, fire management was different from what it is today. The Southeast and Western portions of the United

States were more prone to fire outbreaks, but small outbreaks weren't necessarily seen as a bad thing. Many landowners in these areas recognized that smaller, regular fires were necessary to remove fuel sources that could otherwise build up and escalate into a potentially extreme fire condition. A new school of thought, however, was growing within the forestry schools, which were influenced by the German approach to fire prevention. The Germans emphasized a scientific and ordered view of management. Proponents of this view stressed that just letting fires burn was a savage approach. To them, this was not forestry or conservation, but simply "destruction." It also impeded a country's ability to keep its timber supply at the highest level. To allow a small tree to burn was akin to extinguishing the light of life in nature.

From the 1930s to the 1970s, forest fire management was codified by the "10 a.m. policy," so-called because fires were to be under control by 10:00 a.m. the next day. This encouraged a fast and all-encompassing fire suppression tactic. Over the years, some objections were raised, but even these were tempered by the idea that so much fuel had now been protected, that to allow the fires to burn again would result in an even bigger disaster. In fact, that is in line with what we now see as an unintended consequence of overaggressive conservation. By limiting the number of tree species that burned, an encroachment of less-fire-tolerant species has now grown where previously it may have been limited. For example, in the Western United States, less-fire-tolerant Douglas fir and Grand fir have taken over swaths of forest normally dominated by more fire-resistant Ponderosa pines. Also, by moving closer to forests and preserving them, people have allowed areas that used to have more frequent, low-intensity fires to become denser with fire-burning fuel. These more intense fires burn more land and are harder to control. They also end up wiping out the seeds of the more fire-resistant tree species, creating a cycle of destruction. And of course, drought conditions in the western United States have only further contributed to the problem. In the end, the cost of fighting these more intense fires has resulted in an increase in fire suppression cost and an increase in the areas burned (see graph below). So now, the forest services are left in a bit of a conundrum. The previous policy of total conservation and suppression has not worked out, and yet to just let nature retake its course will result in even more uncontrollable fires. Newer policies allowing smaller, controlled fires may be the best answer to today's forest fire problem.

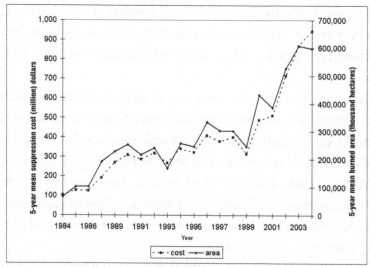

Five-year averages of areas burned by fires greater than 120 ha on US Forest Service land and corresponding suppression costs. From: "Be Careful What you Wish For: The Legacy of Smokey Bear." Donovan G and Brown T. *Front Ecol Environ* 2007; 5(2): 73–79. Courtesy of Geoffrey Donovan.

In 1920, as the current philosophy of forest fighting was taking shape, S.E. White wrote, "In other words, if we try to burn it out now, will we not get a destructive fire? We have caught the bear by the tail—can we let it go?" He cautions that we may have just dug our own hole and now we can't quite get out of it. Ironically, he references a bear like Smokey, but then again, he could he have just as easily said a cobra. Perhaps too much safety can be a bad thing. If we end up protecting something too much that needs a little bit of danger, do we end up in a situation where there is no turning back, where we have done so much to make things safe that it is now unsafe? Maybe a little *controlled* burning here and there is a good thing. In the world of car racing, maybe a *controlled* crash here or there isn't a bad thing, but allowing the crashes to get out control can lead the sport to a reckoning point of no return.

ON MAY 1, 1994, DALE Earnhardt arrived at the Talladega Speedway postrace interview, kissed his wife, and held his daughter in his arms. He looked around at the media, who he knew would ask him what it was like to win his seventh Winston Cup, tying Richard Petty for the most all-time. But first, he wanted to address something else. He began to speak, the thrill of victory still resonating in his voice. The first words out of his mouth preempted the media's questions about his victory. He wanted to take a moment to mention the name Ayrton Senna.

That very same day, the same day Dale tied a major NASCAR record, a tragic loss in the racing world reverberated from across the Atlantic Ocean. In Italy, three-time Formula One world champion and legendary driver Ayrton Senna had been leading the pack in the 1994 San Marino Grand Prix. Live-feed cameras broadcast the race to a worldwide audience. Suddenly, his car spun out of control and crashed into a concrete barrier. Debris flew everywhere, and the world of F-1 Racing came to a screeching halt.

The circumstances leading up to that moment were equally if not more tragic for the safety of racing. The qualifiers for the 1994 San Marino Grand Prix had occurred two days prior to the official race. That year, electronic balance and suspension systems had been done away with, leaving many drivers feeling as if their cars were harder to control. On Friday, April 29, Jordanian driver Rubens Barichello was in a practice lap when his car turned a corner and vaulted through a fence, leaving him suspended upside down and unconscious. His car appeared to literally take off and fly through the air like an airplane. The crashed left him with a broken nose and a broken arm. The next day, on Saturday, April 30, Austrian driver Roland Ratzenberger tried to get the battle with his own rebellious car back under control. During his practice run, he would also lose control of the car and subsequently hit an opposing concrete barrier wall almost head-on. In a shock to all those preparing to race, he suffered a basilar skull fracture and would die that same day. A chill swept over the event.

Ayrton Senna was known not just for his rarefied level of driving, but also for his uncanny ability to control his car in less than favorable conditions. He was a master of racing in the rain. In just his second year of racing in Formula One, while stealthily navigating a wet track, he outmaneuvered every other driver to win his first Grand Prix. Not only did he set himself apart from the crowd with the victory, but he managed to completely lap all but one other driver. Ayrton brought his car to the limit every single race. He would speed so fast into a turn that he and the car would do a little dance as the car teetered between control and chaos. Senna was such a skilled driver that he won his first Formula One world championship title by overcoming a stalled start that placed him 14 cars behind. His comeback, of course, started in the rain. He would go on to win two more world championships before his 32nd birthday.

The day after Ratzenberger's crash, and two days after Barichello's crash, it was race day. The specter of mortality hung like a fog on the racetrack. Several people close to Senna suggested he shouldn't race, including F1's doctor and his close personal friend Prof. Sid Watkins. You have nothing left to prove, he told Senna. Let's just go fishing, he proposed. Yet, despite the fears of those around him, and his own concerns about the safety and temperature-based performance of the cars' tires, Senna decided he would still race. Nicki Lauda pulled Senna aside and lobbied for a return of a drivers' association. Lauda himself was known for his own in-race accident that left him severely burned. Only a few weeks later against the advice of many, he returned to racing, still dealing with blood-soaked bandages on his skin, just to face his rival James Hunt. For years after, Lauda had been a proponent for increased track safety.

The next day, before he went out on the track, Ayrton spent part of the morning talking to the man he battled for most of his career, former teammate and nemesis Alain Prost. Having had a bitter rivalry with Prost, the two of them rarely talked anymore, but that morning things were different. Over breakfast, amidst new safety concerns, the drivers discussed revitalizing the defunct Grand Prix Drivers' Association (GPDA). Senna offered to adopt the chairman role starting after their next race in Monaco. The GDPA would give drivers the voice they lost when the GDPA was disbanded in the 1980s due to conflicts stemming from commercial arrangements and the Formula One Constructors who built the cars. This new plan would reestablish communication between the sanctioning organization (Formula One), the drivers, the commercial entities, and the car constructors.

Finally, it was time to start the race. All the cars lined up in their starting positions, with Senna situated at the head of the pack, a spot he earned as pole position. At 2 p.m., the cars had just finished their warm-up laps and their engines were raring to go, the sound of the engines echoing a swarm of bees. First the four gantry lights flashed red, and then a second later they turned green. Almost immediately, two of the racing cars toward the back of the pack crashed together, sending debris everywhere. Senna, however, was well in front and continued to race. About 15 minutes later, the Brazilian approached the infamous Tamburello curve. He had managed the racetrack turn several times before in this race alone, but this time his car uncharacteristically veered off the track at full speed. Approaching 160 mph, his car slammed sideways into an unprotected concrete wall. The momentum of the crash ricocheted throughout his body. His brain smashed into the walls of his skull. While the medical crew attended to him, including his longtime friend and doctor Prof. Watkins, his body let out a small shudder and sigh. In that moment, it became obvious to Watkins. Ayrton Senna was no longer there. He was brain-dead.

Just days later, still in mourning, the drivers began to band together and demand change. At the next race in Monaco, as Ayrton had planned, the GPDA would be reformatted and include the drivers' voices. The Fédération Internationale de l'Automobile (FIA) responded quickly and introduced changes to the regulations. Even then in Monaco, there was another practice accident. The following day, the FIA president Max Mosley announced the formation of a new Expert Advisory Group. The group would initially consist of Formula One's chief medical advisor and neurosurgeon Prof. Watkins, race director Charlie Whiting, safety delegate Roland Bruynseraede, technical advisor Peter Wright, driver representative Gerhard Berger, and designer representative Harvey Postlethwaite. Demonstrating a true theoretical attempt to avoid the cobra, Charlie Whiting reflected on that moment for the UK's *Independent*: "The important thing was to do the right research because what you sometimes think is the right thing to do intuitively often turns out not to be the case." The advisory group would take a multifaceted approach, focusing on improving both car and cockpit designs, better crash barriers, and safer racetrack configurations with less dangerous corners and more room for car runoff. There would not be another tragedy in Formula One for twenty years, and the global popularity of the sport would continue to rise even as the safety measures would take effect. The advisory group would also continue to employ the services of top-name drivers and car designers throughout the years. Together, the competing interests of the organization worked together to solve the problem.

Back across the ocean, and one month shy of the 7-year anniversary of Senna's death, Dale Earnhardt was in his final lap of the Daytona 500. It was February 2001, and the man nicknamed the "Intimidator" because of his aggressive driving skills was coming up on turn three. In the previous nine months, three NASCAR drivers had died of basilar skull fractures. Ayrton Senna had also suffered a basilar skull fracture. Dale, however, wasn't one to fear death. In fact, Dale was a sort of grim reaper himself on the track. The appearance of his black-clad #3 car suddenly appearing in the rearview mirror would send shivers down even an experienced driver's spine. He would demand any other driver's focus, because if he was behind you, you were going to get hit. He would punch at you like an impatient shark. Either move or get eaten. If there wasn't a hole in the traffic, or the paved track wasn't wide enough, Dale didn't care. He made his own hole or drove off the track to get around you. If you tapped him with your car on one lap, he hit you twice on the next loop. He had an icy-cold stare that was only matched by his no-nonsense attitude. He loved to be side by side, hitting and pounding with another driver. He thrived on testing people and the cars they drove to see what they were made of.

Dale's biggest adversary, however, might not have been another driver. It was the Daytona 500 race. It was no small opponent and was the highest-paying race on the circuit. It was the first to be televised and was even dubbed "The Super Bowl of NASCAR." Dale's first tango with the Florida racetrack was in 1978, when he was left wanting. Throughout the 1980s, despite a very successful racing career, he continued to suffer several more losses at Daytona. Then, in 1990, Dale found himself with a 40-second comfortable lead over the other drivers. He was a quarter of a lap away from that elusive Daytona victory. He turned the corner in his car, where some debris from a previous blowup was on the track. In the blink of an eye, a piece of the debris went through one of his tires and sidelined his car. His first Daytona victory was within sight and he had to pull up short again and it grated on him. It was a rare moment of on-track emotion for the stone-cold competitor. Dale would have the damaged tire mounted on the wall of his garage as a reminder of that fateful day.

The next few visits to Daytona would result in more losses and yet another last-minute loss in 1992 to Dale Jarrett. In a continued twist of ill-fate, Earnhardt was battling for victory on the same racetrack again in 1997 with 12 laps left to go. He was holding the second spot when his car made contact with the wall. Sliding off the wall, the car behind him flipped Earnhardt's car upside down. His car was hit a second time while upside down before flipping back onto its tires. Gradually, he brought #3 to the infield. The on-field crew was hitching the car up to be towed when Dale, still in the ambulance, noticed the tires were still full of air and the wheels aligned straight. So he told the team to unload his car. He had someone test if it could restart, and then he drove it right over to the pit and began barking orders. There, his crew literally taped his car back together, including reattaching the detached spoiler and bumper. Like a cowboy who got knocked off the saddle, the "Man In Black" got back up on his horse and rode it to the finish line.

The next year was 1998. At the Daytona 500, Dale had just met a huge fan name Wessa Miller, who was overcoming a disabling condition known as spina bifida. This young lady gave Earnhardt a lucky penny, and Dale quickly saw to it that the good luck charm was glued onto his dashboard so he could see it during the race. It must have worked, because later that afternoon, on his 20th try, after a long and successful racing career, Earnhardt finally won his first Daytona 500. The "Intimidator," who some say had a hidden heart of gold, pumped his fist toward the clear blue Florida sky. That wonderful day, every crewman on the track lined up to shake the legendary racecar driver's hand. To this day, Wessa's lucky penny still sits in Earnhardt's 1998 Daytona 500-winning car just below the oil gauge.

Just three years later, Dale found himself back on the track at Daytona, but this time he was sponsoring two other cars—those of Michael Waltrip and his own son, Dale Earnhardt, Jr. For the first time, at 160mph, Dale the veteran found himself driving not as the aggressor, but as the defensive player protecting his two teammates. In what might have been considered a passing of the torch, Dale's racing strategy ushered in Waltrip and Jr. into the number 1 and 2 spots of the day. Dale the elder worked that day not to beat his nemesis the Daytona 500, but rather to hold the entire track at bay so the other two cars could maintain their lead and coast to victory. Dale managed this strategy until the very final lap.

On this particular day in 2001, most of the audience's eyes were on Victory Lane, where Dale's teammate Michael was celebrating his first NASCAR victory. Michael's brother was announcing, and joy filled him as he watched his brother speed across the finish line. But soon his eyes and then everyone's collective attention began to shift to somewhere else on the Daytona 500 track. There was a sense in the air that something was wrong. Two cars had hit the wall on the fourth and final turn, and from the looks of it, the cars belonged to #36 Kenny Schrader and #3 Dale Earnhardt. Schrader had been battling a pack of cars when Earnhardt's car, which had been at the head of the trailing pack, made contact with that of another driver, Sterling Marlin.

The Intimidator's car shot up the side of the track and into the wall. Schrader tried but couldn't avoid hitting Earnhardt's car, impaling his car on the passenger side. Schrader hit Earnhardt at the dreaded "one o'clock angle," which is important, because in the NASCAR stock cars, there isn't anything to the right of the steering wheel to catch the driver's head as it whips forward. So, with Earnhardt feeling the impact of the crash, both cars locked up. Together, they bounced off the wall before spinning around and sliding in a T-formation right through the other cars and onto the infield.

Kenny Schrader emerged out of his yellow M&M's-sponsored Pontiac and had run over to Dale's black Chevy. What Schrader saw took his breath away. His longtime friend was slumped over in the car, unconscious. Something inside Kenny told him Dale wasn't waking up. Kenny rushed off the field and gave a quick interview, pale as death. Earnhardt was rushed off to the hospital, where doctors would explain he, like several ill-fated drivers before him, suffered a basal skull fracture. It proved to be a fatal blow to Dale and a near-fatal blow to NASCAR.

In the 1990s, NASCAR teams had begun to work with engineers on building stronger and faster cars. The stiffer cars improved race times, but they also gave less during crashes. As a result, drivers began to receive a greater brunt of the crash impact. Greater forces experienced by the drivers is what many people think led to the increased number of deaths in NASCAR. It didn't take long for Earnhardt's death to trigger a safety overhaul of NASCAR. One thing NASCAR had been working on was creating more give in the concrete barriers that lined the track so at least some energy would be absorbed by the walls and not the car. The other thing that was already being actively discussed was the HANS device.

The "Head and Neck System" was designed to help stabilize the driver, but before Earnhardt's death, it was optional. Some drivers chose to use it. Earnhardt did not. He called the six-point restraint a "noose" and objected to how it limited his vision and ability to look around. It would make it difficult to get out of the car quickly, as well. He also resisted the use of a full-face helmet for the same visual reason. In his mind, he walked away from all his previous crashes, and tightening up the driver wasn't the answer. After a while, the engineers who showed off the device knew they weren't welcome in Earnhardt's garage, and so they just stopped trying to talk to him about it. Their experience was far from unique. Dale only wanted to hear what Dale wanted to hear. On or off the track, Dale let people know who was the boss. You either did things his way, or you got out of the way.

The fact that Earnhardt suffered a basilar skull fracture leaves some mystery as to how he actually died. A fracture at the base of the skull could occur from blunt trauma to the head, one in which additional restraints may have limited the impact. However, there is some research that if the body is restrained but the head keeps moving, then the force of the head trying to come off the body can also cause a basilar skull fracture. When the base of the skull breaks, the foramen magnum also fractures. The foramen magnum is a hole at the base of the skull where the brainstem connects the brain to the spinal cord. A fracture through the foramen magnum can be deadly by injuring the part of the brainstem that controls breathing, or it can tear apart the vertebral or spinal arteries.

Since NASCAR and some drivers were already experimenting with the HANS device, it didn't take long for most of the drivers to adopt it. Their initial resistance was largely based on the idea that the injury "couldn't happen to them," but once Dale died, that attitude changed. If it could happen to the immortal Dale Earnhardt, then maybe they should reconsider their viewpoint. In response, the NASCAR drivers began to use either the HANS device or an alternative called the Hutchens device. Technically, though, NASCAR didn't officially require head-restraint devices until October of 2001 after Blaise Alexander, a driver in the Automobile Racing Club of America (ARCA), a Midwest-based sanctioning body for stock car auto racing, also died of a basilar skull fracture.

The story of Dale's death did not stop there. Significant controversy would ensue as to how Dale actually died. The autopsy found the following clues: 1) a 2.5cm x 1.0cm abrasion over the chin; 2) a similar-sized abrasion over the left collar-bone; 3) a larger abrasion over the left hip; 4) superficial abrasions over the right hip; and 5) a large purple-red area over the abdomen. Five days after the fateful crash, having been presented with evidence by NASCAR, Dr. Steve Bohannon, the chief emergency doctor at Daytona International Speedway, announced that a broken lap belt had allowed Earnhardt to be thrust forward and to the right. His head moved far enough forward that his chin struck the steering wheel, bending the wheel itself, and leading to a basilar skull fracture. The first paramedics to get to the car, however, stated that while the seat belts were loose, they were not broken.

Due to the three related deaths in NASCAR over the previous year at the Florida speedway, the *Orlando Sentinel* had published an investigative series of articles on safety prior to the Daytona 500. With Earnhardt's death still under controversy, the paper wished to pursue an even deeper investigation. Following a court battle, Dr. Barry Myers, a Duke University expert in crash injuries, was appointed to perform an independent investigation. After reviewing the evidence, Myers said that while Earnhardt's head did whip forward into the steering wheel, the driver likely died because his head and neck were not held securely in place. The considerable forces that occur from an unrestrained head and neck during a high-speed frontal crash could kill anyone. The paper had also recruited Dr. Philip Villanueva, a University of Miami neurosurgeon who had come to the same conclusion as Myers based on the autopsy report. But to be certain, Villanueva wanted to examine the autopsy photos.

This is the point at which Earnhardt's death reverberated not just across racing, but also into the courts regarding ideas about freedom of the press. Prior to Dale's death, Florida had what was considered some of the most open public records access laws, ensuring that the state's citizens and media outlets could examine the state's governmental actions. A sportswriter for the *Orlando Sentinel*, Ed Hinton, had petitioned to get copies of the racecar driver's autopsy records and photos. Normally, these were considered public documents in the state of Florida. However, at the urging of Dale's widow, a county judge had placed these under seal. A court battle ensued, which was resolved when

Governor Jeb Bush and the Florida legislature passed the Earnhardt Family Protection Act. With the law, the government hoped to prevent public dissemination of "a photograph or video or audio recording of an autopsy" in order to shield family members from emotional distress.

The law and court ruling, however, were not without controversy. Some critics felt the real motivation of the governor was to protect NASCAR from public criticism regarding its failure to require a head-and-neck restraint system. If true, it could translate into economic misfortune for the company. Others saw a potential unintended consequence that would interfere with the investigation and reporting of controversial deaths by the media. This would set up a conflict between a family's constitutional right of privacy and the public's right to access public records and documents. According to the text of the law, if the media wanted access to these documents, they had to prove that the public's right to know was a "good cause." Otherwise, investigators could be denied access if a judge ruled there was not "good cause" to access the records. As a way to limit controversy, some critics of the law have the idea of mending it to focus specifically on preventing the copying of autopsy photos. This would still allow independent investigators access to review what many consider public records as long as they reviewed the documents under supervised and secure conditions.

While an appeal regarding the Earnhardt case was denied by the US Supreme Court, a similar case did indeed make its way up to the highest court in the land. In that case, a California attorney sought death scene photos of an apparent suicide of a longtime Clinton family lawyer and advisor. The plaintiff attorney, a known political opponent of Bill Clinton, had sought the photos under the premise that foul play might have been involved and that the person in question had not committed suicide, as multiple investigations had concluded. Justice Anthony Kennedy ruled that "family members have a personal stake in honoring and mourning their dead and objecting to unwarranted public exploitation." The Earnhardt family had supported this decision, as did the Bush administration at the time. Free press advocates, however, frowned at the now-federal-level ruling that continued to hinder the public's right to know. Some areas where this law could be used to block access to the public, they would point out, might include investigations into 9/11 or soldiers' deaths. In essence, the case involved the application of an exemption due to privacy of the often-cited federal Freedom of Information Act. A similar controversy existed after the Challenger space shuttle explosion when the *New York Times* wished to obtain recordings from cabin right before the launch. The families of the astronauts sided with NASA on blocking the tapes from being released. The court found that the *New York Times* lawsuit was not justified following NASA's release of a transcript instead of the actual audio recordings.

One of the key players in the legal battle surrounding the Earnhardt autopsy photos was Jon Mills, who is now a University of Florida dean emeritus and law professor. He was the attorney retained by Dale Earnhardt Inc. and Theresa Earnhardt in regard to the autopsy photos. What gave him relevant prior experience was that he had represented Giovanni Versace's family after the fashion designer's death in Miami. The day after Dale died, Jon was contacted by Dale Earnhardt Inc. He had worked with some of the corporation's attorneys previously, so it was an easy choice for them. Because he had been through the process, what sticks out most in the law professor's mind is that the Dale Earnhardt Family Protection Act could be enacted retroactively, meaning it could be applied to cases that took place before the law was approved. That is rare for bills and the legal system. In his personal experience, the Earnhardt Act actually came into play several times afterward, as well. One of his most notable encounters after the bill was passed occurred when he represented the family of Sea World trainer Dawn Brancheau. His legal assistance was sought to prevent the video recording of her death being widely circulated. What ended up being important in that case was that the medical examiner actually described the video in his autopsy report, and therefore the judge ruled that the information included in the report, like the NASA transcript, was enough to satisfy the public interest and still respect the victim's family.

Much like Len Bias's death was a catalyst for change in the law, so was Dale Earnhardt's. Mills sees it like this. If Dale weren't a famous

NASCAR driver, "Would it have been House Bill number one? I don't think so." Perhaps we shouldn't wait for these events to happen on a big stage before we act with legislation. He uses the analogy of dangerous intersections to illustrate his point: "We often put stoplights at intersections only after the death of the driver."

While the Earnhardt family fought in the courtroom, NASCAR fought in the arena of public opinion. The company couldn't risk, nor did it want, any more drivers dying, so the safety overhaul didn't stop with neck restraints. NASCAR wanted to redesign the whole stock car. This is where the cobra really made its way onto the NASCAR track. Safety is always the top priority, but NASCAR took that mantle and went ahead with a redesign of the stock car with minimal input from key voices. The decision was made much to the chagrin of the racing teams, drivers, and fans. The broad overhaul in the name of safety saved drivers but may have almost killed NASCAR.

NASCAR spent the next five years developing the next generation of stock car safety. Their new plan centered on the concept that all racing cars would be based off the same template, something nicknamed "the claw." The claw would fit over the cars as a standardized design and limit the changes different car manufacturers could make to each team's cars. The newer car would also have a reduced dependence on the physics of aerodynamics. The windshield would be more upright and increase the drag, and the bumper would be more box-like, which would catch more air. Both of these effects would combine to slow the car down. It would also make it easier for cars to pass one another on the track.

Many people, even nonrace fans, have heard of "drafting." Drafting occurs when a car in the lead pierces the air in front of it. Air moves over the top of the car and is deflected by the spoiler in the back. If another car trails close enough, then the same air continues to be deflected around the second car and sucks it forward. As a result, both cars can travel faster than either car can go by itself. However, if the lead car turns, the trailing car has to deal with a sudden change in the air pattern. Drafting up to that point usually creates less of a downforce on the front tires of the trailing car, so the tires are less stable.

This can then create what is called the "aero push." When the lead car turns, the trail car driver may suddenly lose control and be "pushed" toward the walls, causing a spectacular crash, much to the delight of fans. But it also meant long lines of cars drafting rather than racing side by side, something NASCAR hoped would increase with the Car of Tomorrow design.

From a safety standpoint, the driver's seat was moved four inches to the right side, and the roll cage was moved three inches toward the back. The overall size of the car was also increased by a couple of inches. This would allow more space to be built into the car that could collapse on impact. This is known as a larger "crumple zone" and would absorb more of the energy before it got to the driver. The newer cars also had to weigh a minimum of 3,400 pounds (1,542 kilograms), with at least 1,625 pounds (737 kilograms) of the weight on the right side of the car—the side that most often hits the wall. NASCAR introduced the car officially on the track in 2007. Driver Kyle Busch won the first race using the Car of Tomorrow and then promptly declared that it "sucked." He was also quoted at the victory lane as saying, "I'm glad we could come out of here with a victory, but I still can't stand to drive these things. They're terrible." The Car of Tomorrow would suffer some initial design setbacks, as well. Initially, the front part of the car could run into the back tire of another car and puncture it. The safety foam used on the sides of the car actually caught fire and engulfed the driver's cockpit with smoke. That same foam would also shear off during crashes and leave debris all over the racetrack. These issues, however, would be resolved.

One issue that didn't seem to resolve was the attempt to reduce the aero-push on the trailing car. To some drivers, the redesign actually had the opposite effect. In 2008, Kyle Busch reiterated why he disliked the car, stating that coming up behind another car was like "hitting a wall of air." Several drivers complained that it felt like they had to "relearn" driving strategies at the same racetracks they had been racing at their whole careers. To those watching the races, it became more difficult for drivers to slingshot around the cars in front of them, which in essence limited the exciting back-and-forth maneuvers NASCAR fans had come to love. Racing also became more of a "team sport," similar to how Formula One had evolved. Rather than one guy trying to beat everyone out on the track, drivers would have to coordinate over their radios to swap positions as they made their way around the loops.

But perhaps what really irked fans was the way the new cars looked. They all looked the same: big, boxy, and generic. Some fans couldn't even tell the cars apart. All the distinguishing curves and features were gone, and in their place were just identifying insignia. In fact, NASCAR Chairman and CEO Brian France looked back on the Car of Tomorrow as his biggest failure, most of which he attributed to the lack of unique manufacturer identities. According to the *Detroit Free Press*, France remarked, "We just didn't get the collaboration we needed to get from the industry, the owners, the drivers, the engineers and car manufacturers. They had a voice, but they didn't have a loud enough voice." Perhaps he might have envisioned a committee with more diverse seats at the table, similar to the F1 Expert Advisory Group following Senna's death.

To those who were looking for a more competitive race, there is some solace in statistics. During the five full seasons that the Car of Tomorrow was on the track, there were at least a dozen different winners in each of the 36-race schedules. The last two seasons saw 33 different drivers cruise into Victory Lane. But to the core of NASCAR fans, that's not what they wanted to see. They wanted to see cars they recognized with drivers they knew, so they could cheer them to victories. The cars were, without a doubt, safer, but fans could hardly cheer for their favorite American manufacturer rivalry between Ford or Chevrolet cars. That same year, the American-only barrier was broken when the Toyota Camry was introduced into the stock car racing mix. NASCAR also looked to branch out beyond its core "All-American" audience and rebrand itself. While more traditional states were closing down racetracks, racing executives were pushing expansion into less traditional, but perhaps more fickle, markets like Las Vegas and Southern California.

Since that time, NASCAR has seen a steady decline in ratings year by year.

Bloomberg did an analysis of speedway attendance, and while there are some peaks from 2007 to 2008, there is an obvious decline after 2008, which is when the Car of Tomorrow was introduced.

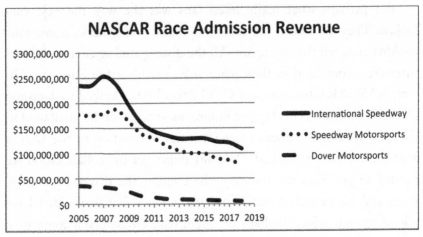

NASCAR Race Admissions Revenue. Source: Bloomberg, company reports.

SportsMediaWatch.com has also compiled a similar trend by compiling ratings data of NASCAR's biggest race of the year, the Daytona 500. Despite the 2006 Daytona 500 attracting the sixth-largest live global TV audience of any sporting event that year with 20 million viewers, NASCAR could not capitalize after that and would subsequently suffer a ratings decline.

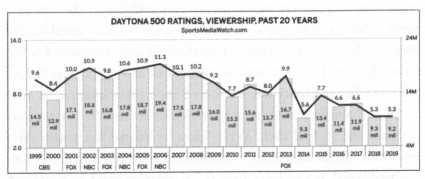

Courtesy of SportsMediaWatch.com.

Today, Aytron Senna's legacy organization, Formula One, is in the midst of its own battle between identity and safety. Now, albeit maybe a bit late in our story, might be a good time to differentiate Formula One racing and culture from that of NASCAR. Formula One has its roots in the wealthy playboys of Europe, while NASCAR has been a traditional American sport born from bootleggers. Formula One employs a traditional open cockpit style with shorter races and quicker snaking turns, whereas NASCAR showcases enclosed cars with longer, looping races. Formula One cars are also lighter and faster. They are made for a sprint versus NASCAR's marathon.

Following the Senna tragedy, Formula One racing had not had a death on the course for twenty years until a tragic incident involving Jules Bianchi at the 2014 Japanese Grand Prix. Bianchi had been racing under very wet conditions brought on by the approaching Typhoon Phanfone. Daylight was also fading, and as the French racer came around a corner, Bianchi lost control of his car and veered onto the run-off area on the outside of the curve. Suddenly, he flew underneath the rear of a tractor crane that was in the process of removing a car that had also spun out of control and crashed in the same area just one lap prior. Partly in response to Bianchi's death as well as another head-injury related deaths in IndyCar, Formula One mandated that all cars be fitted with a halo device. In a nod to NASCAR's Car of Tomorrow shell, it was decreed that the new device be formed by one part that was made by a single company so all the cars would have to fit it the same way.

Since the mandatory ruling, the halo device has divided the Formula One community. Longtime fans point out F1 racing should maintain its identity as an open-cockpit sport. Some drivers say the device restricts their vision. Others say it makes it difficult so see their favorite drivers. It may even hamper drivers getting in and out of the cars easily. The Mercedes team boss Toto Wolff was quoted as saying, "If you give me a chainsaw, I would take it off." He did continue, though, by following up with "I think we need to look after the driver's safety, but we need to come up with a solution that simply looks better."

His sentiments echoed several of the original criticisms of NASCAR's Car of Tomorrow.

This may be Formula One's safety Cobra Effect if it does not listen to its drivers and designers as it did so well following Senna's death. It's also worth noting that this Formula One controversy comes on the heels of another Cobra Effect aimed at increasing racing excitement. In 2016, Formula One introduced a new rule with barely two weeks' notice. A new qualifying system would be enacted where the slowest car was to be eliminated every 90 seconds. However, rather than increasing fan and racing excitement, the new ruling resulted in an empty track for much of the qualifiers and was scrapped after just two races.

With the Car of Tomorrow, NASCAR addressed a much-needed increase in safety but as a result lost some of its identity. And now with the halo controversy, will Formula One be undoing what had been many successful years of cooperation between the sanctioning body, drivers, and designers in its own quest for safety? Will the halo be Formula One's Car of Tomorrow?

7

Duk-koo Kim and Boxing's
Biggest Tragedy

THERE ARE SEVERAL UPSIDES TO bicycling. It is a healthy and environ-
mentally conscious mode of transportation. It's pretty cost-effective.
And some of the happiest cities on Earth have adopted it as a primary
mode of travel. And yet, lurking like a cobra in the shadows, there
is an element of danger. Whether it's a pig-tailed yonug girl cruising
along the neighborhood street or a bike messenger weaving in and out
of rush-hour traffic, severe bicycle accidents can result in life-altering
injuries. Fortunately, there is some protection. In the United States,
evidence has shown that bicycle helmets can reduce the likelihood of
serious head trauma and brain damage by as much as 85 percent. In
this same vein of rider safety, various mandatory helmet laws have been
implemented around the world. Unfortunately, although these laws are
made with the best of intentions, some have had unintended consequences. For an example, let's turn to Australia, where a mandatory
bicycle helmet law aimed at reducing injuries actually ended up making
bicycling less safe.

Before 1991, only about 37 percent of Australian cyclists were
using helmets while riding. Then, in 1991, a law was passed mandating

the use of a bicycle helmet. After the law went into effect, encouraging numbers showed the percentage of riders using a helmet surpassed 80 percent. Since bicycle helmets protect the head, lawmakers naturally assumed that an increase in helmet usage would coincide with a decrease in the number of cyclist head injuries. Researchers in Western Australia, however, found quite a different story. They compared the percentage of head injuries in cyclists that were admitted to the hospital after an accident before and after the mandatory helmet law was introduced. What they found was that there didn't seem to be any significant changes once the law went into effect. In the graph below, you can see there already was an overall declining trend for the two decades before the helmet law was introduced. Then, after the law was introduced in 1991, there didn't seem to be any further decline, and in fact, there was even a small spike around 1995.

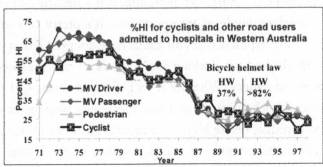

Percent of Head Injuries (%HI) of Patients Admitted to the Hospital in Western Australia. %HW = Percent Wearing Helmets. Image Courtesy of Dr. Dorothy L Robinson.

A similar analysis was done in New Zealand, where the same researchers plotted graphs of the percentage of adults and the percentage of school-age children who used bicycle helmets. They then placed lines on the same graphs showing head injury rates in adults and in children. What you see is an obvious spike in the percentage of adults wearing helmets, as the law intended. But what isn't apparent is a corresponding decrease in adult head injuries. Helmet wear goes up, but the rate of head injuries didn't change.

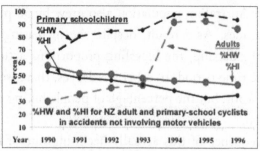

Percent of Primary New Zealand Schoolchildren
and Adults Wearing Helmets (%HW) and Percent
with Head Injuries (%HI). Image Courtesy of Dr.
Dorothy L Robinson.

In another study, researchers wanted to know how many people were actually on bicycles in Western Australia before and after the helmet law was enacted. To get this data, automatic counters were set up in the bike lanes of two bridges over the Swan River in Perth, Western Australia. These counters logged the number of cyclists using the bike lanes from October through December. In 1991, before the helmet law was enacted, a total of 16,326 riders was logged. These numbers were compared with the same months in 1992, 1993, and 1994. What the researchers found was that there was a steady decline in the number of cyclists using these bike lanes, leading to a low of 10,701 in 1994. This represented a decline of 35 percent in bicycle ridership. Before the helmet laws went into effect, census data had shown that the number of Australians cycling to work was increasing from 1976 to 1986. This trend continued up until 1991, when the helmet laws were introduced. Following 1991, this number decreased in the states with helmet laws and increased in the states without enforced helmet laws.

Recent data trends seem to show an increase in the total number of bicyclists in Australia even after the helmet laws went into effect. However, some academics and statisticians have held their hands up in protest. They pointed out that if one were to take into consideration the growth of Australia's total population during that time, the increase in ridership may actually not be real. For example, between 1986 and 2006, the number of bicyclists increased by about 20 percent.

However, the Australian population also grew by 58 percent during those two decades. As a result, despite the increasing trend in the graph of total ridership, the bicycling proportions actually declined over that same time period. In other words, yes, there were more people biking to work, but the percentage of people biking to work actually went down.

One consequence of this actually declining rate of bicycle ridership may be an associated increase in injury risk. Bicycling has been shown to be safer when there are greater numbers of cyclists on the road. Injury rates appear to be lower when more people are bicycling. This pattern has been consistent across communities of varying size. Researchers think this is less likely due to the actions of the bicyclists themselves, and more to the reactions of motorists due to the presence of increased numbers of cyclists. There is also some newer research that suggests drivers will actually pass closer to a bicycle rider if the rider is wearing a helmet.

Changes in behavior when a helmet is involved isn't limited to just the person behind the wheel of a car. There is some evidence that wearing a bicycle helmet may actually increase the risky behavior of cyclists, at least in a laboratory setting. Researchers from the Department of Psychology at the University of Bath performed an experiment on 80 participants between the ages of 17 and 56. In clinically approved subterfuge, the subjects were told they were participating in an eye-tracking experiment. In the actual variable being studied, the eye-tracking devices were secured onto their heads with either a bicycle helmet or a baseball cap.

The participants then played a computerized game in which they had to press a button to inflate a balloon on the screen in front of them. Each time they pressed the button, the balloon inflated further and they would earn a fictional amount of currency. The balloons were set to randomly burst. If the balloons popped, the participants would lose their earnings. They could also stop at any point and bank any of their accrued game money. Each participant had the chance to complete 30 balloon-inflating trials.

After all the data were collected, the researchers analyzed it to answer the question of whether there was a difference in risky behavior between those who wore a helmet and those who wore a baseball cap. What the researchers found was surprising. When a subject wore a bicycle helmet, they scored significantly higher on both risk taking and sensation seeking. They were more willing to take risks and inflate the balloon, losing fake currency be damned! What is particularly head-scratching is that wearing a bicycle helmet in this situation versus just a baseball cap would have any effect on how someone acts. All they were doing was inflating a computerized balloon, so there would seem to be no perceived benefit by wearing a bicycle helmet for this type of activity. And yet, according to the data, the effect was statistically real.

At this point, we should mention the name Sam Peltzman, who is a professor emeritus at the Booth School of Business of the University of Chicago. He has spent a large part of his career looking at the interface between the public sector and the private economy. In the 1970s, his career path took him to the automobile industry. It was there that he developed a hypothesis known as the "Peltzman Effect." In essence, what his theory tells us is that people are more likely to engage in risky behaviors in the face of mandated security measures. Peltzman proposed that safety measures like seat belts and air bags may have unintended and opposite consequences. What could happen, he theorized, is that drivers may feel safer with the added features and therefore may drive with less attention or more aggression, creating a more dangerous environment for vehicular traffic. We might translate this to bike helmet safety. Riders with helmets may feel more "invincible" and bike with less regard for safety. Or, as we have already seen, drivers may feel more comfortable passing closer to cyclists wearing helmets.

Researchers from the University of California Irvine decided to take a step back and look at trends in helmet use and bicycle ridership. First, they identified 21 states that had helmet laws for children under 16. Then they looked at how much of an effect on head injuries the helmet laws had. They concluded there was a benefit to the helmet laws, but upon close statistical scrutiny, it was only about one-third of the size implied by previous studies. So, according to their data, we can say helmet laws can help to reduce injury, especially when it comes to bigger head injuries. But the reason why the effect wasn't as big as previously thought was something similar to what was happening halfway across the world in Australia. The population of bicycle riders had decreased after the laws were put in place. In the United States, there appeared to be a statistically significant reduction in youth bicycling participation of about 4 to 5 percent after the mandatory laws were implemented. As a result, previous calculations had failed to take into account the effective proportions of riders wearing helmets.

So, if we at least take things at face value, we can say that bicycle helmets are, overall, a good thing. They can make serious head injuries less serious. However, what does become questionable is the actual beneficial effect of governments mandating the wearing of bicycle helmets. If the goal we set for ourselves is to promote safety, but the research suggests that bicycle helmet laws reduce the safety of numbers, may promote more risky behavior, and isn't as great as we thought, then we might have to wonder if the Australian helmet laws made things more unsafe in the name of safety. A cobra snake in a bicycle helmet would be an odd sight, but perhaps it best illustrates the conundrum of the situation. Trying to overregulate something can end up making it more unsafe. To see this in sports, we just have to look at the world of boxing.

"EITHER HE DIES, OR I die". These were the words Korean boxer Duk-koo Kim uttered to his wife foreshadowing his now-infamous fight. They reflected his macabre view of the upcoming bout with American boxing champion Ray "Boom Boom" Mancini. When Kim left his home country in 1982 for the Las Vegas matchup, the monumental importance of the fight, not only for his career, but also for his family, loomed over him. His fiancée, Young-mi, was pregnant, and the young couple was expecting their first son. Yet, while the light of a new life grew inside his wife, the specter of mortal combat impregnated everything Duk-koo Kim did. Before he left Seoul, Kim had a carpenter rig up a mock coffin. He said he would use the vessel of death to bring back Mancini after the fight. Unimpressed with his bravado, his trainer stomped the coffin to pieces and shoved the remnants of death under the boxing ring. Still, Kim's obsession with the fatality of the fight continued.

The city itself seemed a contrast between life and death. "I remember when we landed in Las Vegas for the fight," his trainer, Kim Yoon-Gu, recalled to Agence France-Presse in 2012. "The city was all lit up at night. It was like landing on a garden of flowers in the desert." Once in Las Vegas, Kim settled into Caesars Palace, where the Roman history of grand gladiatorial battle imbued the atmosphere. Later, while in his hotel room, Kim was interviewed by Royce Feour of the *Las Vegas Review-Journal*. Feour noticed hand-written Korean characters on the lampshade by the fighter's bed and asked the young warrior what the letters meant. The interpreter informed him that Kim had neatly written upon the lampshade the dire warning, "Live or Die."

In another interview approaching the fight, Ralph Wiley of *Sports Illustrated* asked the Korean combatant how his chin was—a reference to his ability to take Manicini's punishment. After a series of exchanges with the interpreter, Wiley grabbed his own jaw with his fingers and moved it side to side to illustrate his question. Seeing this, the fighter's expression suddenly changed. "I would like to say he smiled, but it was something else. Scorn," wrote the journalist. "He [Kim] gently touched his jaw with two fingers of his right hand, then without averting his gaze, he reached over and touched the marble window sill with the same two fingers, just as gently. He turned to face the desert. The interview was over." With his gaze lost over the Las Vegas Desert, Kim's mind may have wandered over the long, tough road that brought him so far from home. This road reflected who he was. To understand Kim as both a person and a fighter, you needed to see where he came from.

Kim was born from poverty. From an early age, he became no stranger to overcoming adversity through sheer will. He pushed ever forward, absorbing life's onslaught of punches. His biological father died when Kim was 2 years old. Then, just three years later, his mother left his stepfather when Kim was just 5 years old. It was not a safe home. His stepfather's oldest son had become violent and abusive. Carrying all of their possessions, the small child and his mother fled to a small fishing village called Banam. There, Duk-koo and his mother eventually moved into a thatch-roofed and plywood house owned by the mother's new husband. In a 2012 *New York Times* article, author Mark Kriegel would describe the house as "ramshackle." It included "a partitioned cinderblock structure in the yard [that] served as both an outhouse and a shelter for the family's most valued possession, a cow."

Growing up with a new family, even at an early age, Kim would learn to fight for the pleasure of others. In his journal, he wrote that his new brother would drag him around, forcing him to fight with kids from other villages. The older kids would gather around to enjoy the contests. On the outside, Kim seemed unfazed, but deep inside his soul, he despised them. As a teenager, the young Korean would leave the confines of the small fishing village and move to Seoul. There, in the big city, he lived an even poorer life. He subsisted on odd jobs here and there until one day, he found his way to the Dong-ah boxing gym, which was considered the country's premier boxing gym. It was run by a former fighter named Hyun-chi Kim. Hyun-chi's first impression was that Duk-koo was not fighter material. Yet, Duk-koo persisted. He kept coming back and fighting. Before long, the fellow fighters in the gym took note. He impressed them not with his strength or speed, but rather with his ability to take punishment and keep pressing forward. Before long, Kim rose through the short ranks of Korean boxing. In 1982, with a unanimous decision over his opponent, and some political machinations, Duk-koo suddenly found himself as the World Boxing Association's No. 1 contender.

The man holding the world title belt at that time was Ray "Boom Boom" Mancini, a powerful Italian American boxer many compared to the movie icon Rocky. Ray was a second-generation boxer, and a second-generation "Boom Boom," with his father, Lenny Mancini, sporting the nickname as a boxer up until World War II. Ray grew up in Youngstown, Ohio, among the dying factories of the Rust Belt. In his biographical book, Mark Kriegel describes the young fighter being "cast as the savior of a sport: a righteous kid in a corrupt game, symbolically potent and demographically perfect, the last white ethnic."

In that same year, the players of the NFL had gone on strike. Fans of football were upset and yearned for the controlled action and violence of sport. Seeing an opportunity and eager to shift the fans' attention away from the NFL labor negotiations, CBS decided to air boxing in place of football. Mancini was already garnering the network's highest ratings for a boxer, so CBS officials decided to air a live championship bout. They chose Kim as Mancini's opponent. Although the network bookers didn't know much about Kim, and some had never even heard of him, the few fight clips they saw were of a man who they all agreed was a tough guy. They wanted an opponent for Mancini who wouldn't run. They wanted someone who would stand and exchange with the exciting champion, someone who would not back down and instead would go toe-to-toe with the powerful striker. That was exactly Kim's style.

On November 13, 1982, the two boxers squared off against each other, the irresistible force versus the immovable object. CBS Sports Saturday aired the world title fight live around the world. The broadcast reached millions of households, except that of Kim's own wife. At that time, "going the distance" meant fighting a full 15-round fight. Compared to Kim, Mancini was a much more experienced fighter. In fact, Kim had never gone through a full 15-round fight. Mancini, on the other hand, had already defended his belt several times and come out the victor. Ring announcer Chuck Hull stood in the middle of the outdoor arena and introduced the 23-year-old Kim in the blue corner. The Korean bounced his head around in a spastic tornado of motion, largely to the boos of the pro-American crowd. Then Hull turned his attention to the red corner, where the 21-year-old Mancini was bouncing around in his crimson robe and gleaming title belt. "Boom Boom" shadowboxed behind the announcer and then blew kisses to the crowd with his gloves.

The opening round started with Kim landing a few solid punches, and Mancini answering with bombs of his own. The fighters were temporarily separated by referee Richard Green, and Kim performed a traditional bow before stepping back toward his opponent. From then on, the two fighters would go toe-to-toe each round, with Mancini often unloading a barrage of punches, and the stubborn Korean fighter absorbing the punches and answering with a salvo of his own. There was no doubt that Kim showed he was as strong as the defending champion and could connect just as powerfully. Kim could not be deterred. "Sugar" Ray Leonard, commenting at ringside, would remark that even before this fight, Kim was known for marching straight toward his opponent, sometimes without even throwing a punch. With the Korean leaning in up close, Mancini would fire multiple short, powerful punches. However, after each combination concluded, Ray would move straight backward, rather than to the side. This allowed the Korean to capitalize and attack. Kim also caught Mancini a few times as he wound up to punch standing with his feet flat and wide apart.

At the close of Round 6, chants of "Duk-koo" could be heard intermittently punching above the roar of the crowd, fighting against the larger and more forceful opposing cheers for "Boom Boom." In Round 8, Kim began to dance around and rocked the champion with two big punches right at the sound of the bell. In Round 9, Kim continued to move more on his toes, bringing the fight to the Ohio native. The announcers began discussing whether the rounds should be awarded to Mancini for attacking most of each round, or to Kim, who would wait and wobble the champion at the close of the rounds. Either way, they agreed, this was an even fight. Toward the end of the tenth round, both fighters appeared physically exhausted, Kim resorting to trying to push Mancini's face off of him with both gloves. During the 12th round, Kim began to show further signs of fatigue, losing his balance a few times, but Mancini was unable to put him down. By the end of that round, the crowd was on its feet, cheering on the two mighty gladiators, both their faces bruised and eyes swollen.

During the 13th round, Mancini came running off of his stool and landed 44 straight punches. Despite his legs starting to wobble and loosen, Kim still managed to absorb the blows and mount somewhat of a counterattack. He survived the round, but it was clear that Kim was losing stability on his legs. Between rounds 13 and 14, one of the television announcers, Tim Ryan, remarked, "Duk-koo Kim. You may not have heard of him before—but you will remember him today." Then 19 seconds after the bell into the 14th round, "Boom Boom" connected with two big right hands, dropping the Korean boxer. Kim managed to get to his feet before the count of 10, but seeing the fighter struggling, the referee stopped the fight. Mancini fans rejoiced, but soon an ominous mood quickly fell over the crowd. Kim was being carried out of the ring on a stretcher.

Once out of the arena, the Korean was quickly rushed to nearby Desert Springs Hospital and the operating room. There, neurosurgeon Dr. Lonnie Hammargren removed a blood clot from the Korean boxer's brain. Hammargren, being so close to the boxing mecca, had performed surgery on many boxers' brains before, but even this one, the neurosurgeon said, was "in bad shape." After the surgery, Hammargen told *Sports Illustrated*, "He's very critical, with terminal brain damage. There is severe brain swelling. The pressure will go up and up, and that will be it. He'll die. His pupils have been fixed since he arrived." The doctor followed up with, "They tell me he fought like a lion in the 13th round. Well, nobody could fight like that with a blood clot on his brain."

Tragically, the Korean warrior known for his uncanny ability to absorb punishment and come out the other end attacking met one foe he could not best. His tactic of taking a punch to give a punch eventually was too much of a burden. The trauma to his brain proved fatal. Despite over two hours of surgery to remove a subdural brain hematoma and four days in a coma, the fighter remained down forever. Kim's mother had flown from South Korea to be at his side. She pleaded for him to open his eyes. Eventually, she resigned herself to the loss of her son. Before she left her son's side forever, she agreed to allow American surgeons to transplant his kidneys to needy recipients. She said her true reason for allowing the transplants was "that my son can live forever and have everlasting life in this world." His kidneys were removed at 11:15 p.m., and his death certificate was signed at midnight.

Kim's death sent shockwaves through those connected to him. His fiancée had planned to marry him in a posthumous spiritual wedding to console his spirit but later decided against it. Four months later, Kim's mother would commit suicide by drinking a bottle of pesticide; and less than a year after the fight, the referee, Richard Green, would also take his own life (his motivation is still unclear). Mancini suffered from depression, and many say he was never the same fighter again. The day after the bout, Mancini, his hands still bandaged, prayed for Kim during a mass in the casino ballroom. Even having the legendary Frank Sinatra asking him to stand and be recognized during a celebration, which should have been one of the highlights of his life, left him feeling small and sad. Fans would come up to him in restaurants and ask him what it was like to kill someone. The hype for each of his fights after the tragic event would inevitably loop in the fatal bout. Despite being mortal opponents in the ring, Mancini felt a spiritual connection to Kim outside of the ring. Somehow during the fight, their souls connected. He remarked later that he knew Kim better than anyone else in the world, because he had seen what he was inside. Then, just two weeks later, another pivotal, albeit less immortalized, bout delivered a second stunning blow to the sport of boxing.

On November 24, 1982, heavyweight boxing champion Larry Holmes squared off against a much more inexperienced boxer, Randall "Tex" Cobb. Tex was a wild-haired former kickboxer who, like Kim, was known for an iron chin. During the one-sided fight, veteran referee and two-term Nevada District Court Judge Mills Lane stopped the action to ask Cobb if he was okay. When Cobb replied that he was, Lane asked him, "Do you know where you are?" to which Cobb replied, "I am in Reno, getting the shit kicked out of me." Later, when the title contest was again stopped by Lane to check on Cobb, the referee asked the boxer, "Do you see me?" Cobb then replied, "Yeah. You're white. It's the black guy I'm worried about."

Witty banter aside, the visual of this lopsided bout further catalyzed the demonization of boxing. Iconic sports broadcaster Howard Cosell emphatically described the scene by questioning whether "that referee understands that he is constructing an advertisement for the abolition of the very sport that he is a part of" and that the bout "couldn't have come at a worse time." Soon thereafter, Cosell swore off commentating for boxing due to his grave concerns for the athletes' health, simply saying, "I've had it." Similarly, the editor of the *Journal of the American Medical Association* (*JAMA*) as well as other medical organizations began a crusade against the sport of boxing. It was even labeled as an "obscenity" in a *JAMA* editorial.

Following the debacle, major sponsors began to pull out of deals with CBS and other networks due to the bad publicity associated with boxing. Even Mancini, the reigning champion and fan favorite, was hit in his wallet with the loss of endorsement deals. The times and opinions were changing. While the 1970s viewed boxing as a nobly athletic means to rise out of the poor neighborhoods in America, which was popularized by the movie *Rocky*, the 1980s saw a strong wave of criticism and concern for the athlete's safety and future health. Within a month of the Mancini-Kim bout, the sanctioning body of the fight, the World Boxing Council (WBC), voted unanimously to reduce the number of championship rounds from 15 to 12. Alfredo Lamazont, a WBC spokesman, said recent studies by the WBC had shown more serious injuries in the 13th or 14th rounds of recent fights. The decision by the president of the WBC at the time, José Sulaimán, was heavily criticized. The WBC was taking away valuable minutes of commercials for TV networks and was taking away the drama that occurred during the later "championship" rounds. That's where, fans would describe, the exhausted boxers were really showing what they had inside them by performing purely on heart.

Partly in response to Kim's death, in one of boxing's biggest states, the Nevada State Athletic Commission (NSAC), along with its medical committee chairman Dr. Edwin "Flip" Homansky, lobbied the remaining major boxing sanctioning organizations to permanently change championship bouts from 15 to 12 rounds. In their studies, it wasn't that more deaths occurred in these rounds, but after a careful review of the Kim-Mancini bout and other 15-round contests, it was revealed that in Rounds 13 through 15, the fighters just threw mostly head shots and maintained virtually no defense. Homansky and the NSAC also lobbied to change the number of ring ropes from four to five to prevent fighters from falling out of the ring and through the ropes.

By 1988, all three major boxing organizations agreed to limit the number of boxing rounds, though not without some hesitation and controversy. Opponents to the rule change argued that there were no solid studies showing increased risk after the 13th round and that fatalities were less common in the heavyweight than lighter weight classes. They attribute this to the fact that the lighter weight classes have to cut more weight and are more susceptible to dehydration in later rounds. Boxing fans also pointed to numerous fights that would have had different outcomes had the matches ended at 12 rounds instead of 15. In fact, the controversy was evident the day the WBC announced the rule change. The prevailing opinion of those opposed to the change was echoed by Larry Holmes, the WBC heavyweight champion at the time: "It will cut down on injuries for a lot of fighters, but it will take away from the true champions. A true champion can go 15 rounds."

Yet, Kim's death proved a pivotal moment for change. In 2010, researchers from the University of California San Diego published a retrospective study in the journal *Neurosurgery* where they analyzed boxer deaths secondary to head injury from 1950 to 2007. There were 399 boxer deaths during that time period. The researchers found that there was a significant reduction of professional boxer deaths after 1983, which came after the round rule change. Two-hundred nineteen boxer deaths occurred between 1950 and 1983, but only 120 occurred after 1983. Yet, despite the significanct reduction in boxer deaths, the authors found no significant changes in the number of deaths associated with a knockout (KO). They were unable to identify the round reduction rule as the significant variable to support a decline in KO deaths. In the graph below, you can see no changes in deaths related to KOs in the ring before or after the rule change. In fact, the count even seems to go up for the 10th round from 1983 to 2007.

The authors of the study hypothesized that the decline of deaths after 1983 that were recorded were not due to fewer KO deaths, but rather due to a reduction in exposure to repetitive head trauma (shorter careers and fewer fights), along with increased medical oversight and stricter safety regulations. While the average round for a KO-related death was the 7th round, the majority of KO-related deaths occurred in the 10th round. Another interesting finding of the study was that a higher percentage of deaths occurred in the lower weight classes. While it's obvious heavier boxers deliver more powerful and traumatic punches, they did not lead to more KO deaths. One thought about this is that even though the punches are harder in the heavier weight classes, the bigger, stronger boxers may be able to withstand heavier blows and absorb more with their stronger neck muscles. Lighter fighters may also throw more punches to the head throughout a fight.

Using the same database that the UCSD authors used, and adding in an additional nine years to even the two sides out, shows similar trends. If we look at all recorded boxing deaths for 1950 to 2016, and this time add in amateur fighters, we see the same trend. There appears to be fewer deaths in boxing by KO after the 1983 rule change. We can even add technical knockouts (TKOs) to the total, and the trend persists. Overall, there appears to be fewer deaths in the sport of boxing after 1982. In fact, both groups seem to show the greatest density of boxing deaths in the 1960s. If we use the same broad inclusion criteria of professional and amateur deaths in a bout and break it down by round, we see results similar to the UCSD study. There seems to be very few deaths after the 10th round. The 3rd round seems to be the most deadly, but the second-most deadly round is the 10th. There is even a slight increase in 12th-round boxing deaths after the 1983 rule change.

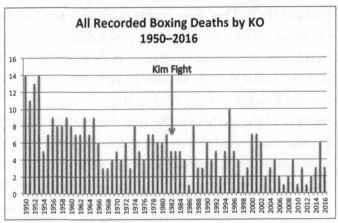

Data Source: The Manuel Velazquez Boxing Fatality Collection,
Courtesy of Joseph Svinth.

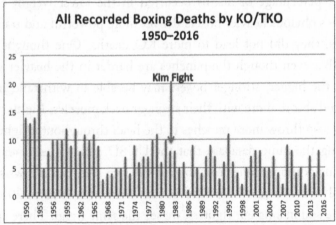

Data Source: The Manuel Velazquez Boxing Fatality Collection,
Courtesy of Joseph Svinth.

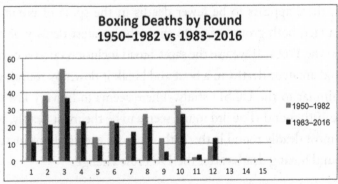

Data Source: The Manuel Velazquez Boxing Fatality Collection,
Courtesy of Joseph Svinth.

Kim's death was not the first and tragically not the last death in boxing. However, it did shed light on the dangers that boxers face, especially when it comes to neurologic trauma. Unfortunately, as the 1980s came to a close, fan interest and corporate sponsorships shifted, and broadcast and journalistic coverage declined. Boxing has since become more of a niche sport. Today, the biggest and strongest athletes and their fans turn to football as their chosen sport of controlled violence as well as the newer sport of mixed martial arts. Therefore, the boxers' battles outside the ring have not been covered as strongly as the effects of concussions on football players have been.

One avenue for change has been congressional legislation. In 1996, Senator and former boxer John McCain cosponsored the Professional Boxing Safety Act of 1996. The Act aimed to establish health, safety, and ethical guidelines for the boxing industry. The objective of the Act was to protect the health and welfare of professional boxers and to ensure that boxing events held in the United States were properly supervised. Under the Act, every professional boxing contest must take place with the approval and supervision of a state boxing commission, every professional boxer must be physically examined before a bout, and copies of the exam must be provided to the local boxing commission. Further, an ambulance and a physician must be present throughout the bout. And finally, every boxer is to be provided with health insurance for injuries sustained during the bout. This act was further enhanced by the Muhammad Ali Boxing Reform Act, whose purpose was to prevent coercive and exploitative abuses of boxers from a contractual and financial standpoint and to increase disclosure within the boxing industry for the ranking of boxers. The legislation created no new federal bureaucracy and imposed no new regulatory mandates on state boxing commissions.

So, while on paper it sounded like a move in the right direction in response to the tragic deaths in the ring, there were some notable loopholes that may have just made the boxing industry worse off. What is not fully understood by most casual fans is that there is no central governing organizational body for boxing, which is in direct contrast to

Major League Baseball (MLB), the National Hockey League (NHL), the National Basketball Association (NBA), and the National Football League (NFL). As a result, boxing and mixed martial arts contests are sanctioned by state athletic commissions in cooperation with the promotional organizations that sell tickets and pay the fighters. The rules governing the contests can vary state by state, or from a state to a Native American casino. Further, some promoters and managers have found ways around the legislation by claiming their services to be that of an "adviser" and thus they can operate under a different set of rules.

The lack of a central regulatory body has made tracking fighters and injuries a challenge as they move from state to state to compete. When a boxer (or MMA fighter) competes, he or she may receive a mandatory suspension due to either an obvious injury that needs to be evaluated by a specialist or a significant enough head trauma that the brain needs time to rest. As a result, the ringside physician may impose a short-term medical suspension. These are reported to the state's sanctioning body where the event took place, but once the athlete leaves the arena, it's very difficult to enforce. Keeping the fighter out of contact while training can only be done by someone in the gym. And unlike a broken bone in a splint or cast, a concussion isn't something you can see. A medical suspension may follow them, but without a centralized database, it becomes difficult for another state to be made aware of the suspension, partly due to patient privacy laws. Thus, a fighter may end up fighting in another state, or on independent Native American soil at a casino, before a medical suspension expires. This is often less of an issue with a big-name fighter and more of an issue with the journeyman whose sole job is to be an "opponent" for an up-and-coming fighter.

Other issues that have come up are the abuse of performance-enhancing drugs (PEDs) and the practice of cutting weight before a fight. Testing for PEDs requires a system in which fighters can be monitored in and out of competition. Coordination of this requires time, money, and personnel that many states do not have. Further, abuses in the system happen and can be masked with Therapeutic Use Exemptions

(TUEs). A fighter may take anabolic steroids, which reduce the body's natural production of testosterone, and then stop taking the steroids before testing. During this time, the anabolic steroids may leave the body or be masked by other substances, and when the athlete's testosterone level is tested, it is found to be low. This is then used as justification for someone with a TUE to legally use testosterone. There are even cases where big-name promotions have approached states and asked for fighters to be allowed to use TUEs, and when those requests were denied, the promotions either took the event to another country or state, or, when threatened with the loss of revenue from the event, the states acquiesced.

Cutting weight before events is also a known dangerous strategy, but nevertheless it persists. Fighters are matched up in weight classes to ensure fair fights. Their weight is usually checked approximately 24 hours before the event. If the fighters don't make weight, then they face fines or miss an opportunity for an official championship fight. And if the fans paid for an official championship fight, then it's in the best financial interest of the promotion to make sure there is enough time to make weight. Unfortunately, many fighters will cut weight too quickly and can end up in the hospital or even die from kidney or other organ failure. And to make matters worse, when fight night does come around, pretty much none of the boxers or MMA fighters actually fight at the weight at which they weighed in.

In 2013, a research group from Appalachian State University published a study in the *Journal of Strength and Conditioning Research*. In the study, the authors looked at 40 professional mixed martial arts fighters. First, they analyzed how much the fighters weighed during weigh-ins and then again 22 hours later for fight night. They also determined how dehydrated they were by measuring the specific gravity of their urine. Specific gravity is a measure of how dense a liquid is compared to water. Winemakers and beer brewers actually use the same measurement to predict the level of alcohol and fermentation at various stages. What the authors of the MMA study found was that, on average, the MMA fighters gained about 3.5 kg (7.7 pounds) between weigh-ins and fight night the next day. Some gained an average of 5.5 kg (12 pounds) or more in the 22 hours before their matches. Further, using urine-specific gravities, they determined that 39 percent of the fighters on fight night were significantly or, even worse, seriously dehydrated.

Another study done in California looked at the weight-class differences of professional boxers and MMA fighters between weigh-ins and the actual fights that took place. The study was performed under the direction of California athletic commissioner, and former professional fighter, Andy Foster as well as ringside physician Paul Wallace (the author of this book was involved in the analysis). It included 387 MMA fighters and 334 boxers. What the results showed was that the average weight gain was 11.74 pounds for MMA fighters and 9.73 pounds for boxers. Results revealed that 81.9 percent of MMA fighters and 87.4 percent of boxers jumped at least one weight class. Furthermore, 36.4 percent of MMA fighters and 62.8 percent of boxers jumped at least two weight classes. Finally, only 42.6 percent of MMA fighters and 32.9 percent of boxers actually fought at the same weight class as their opponents. In order to combat the yo-yo effect of weight cutting, some states have begun to institute weight-gain limits, and post-weigh-in IV rehydration has been banned. But without a central authority, there is no standardization, and rules and processes regarding weight cutting continue to vary by state.

Ringside physicians and some athletic commissions have continued to work together for the benefit of the health and safety of fighters, but unfortunately, until there is a central organization to help run the sports of boxing and mixed martial arts, many of these problems will persist. Legislation such as the Ali Act has the right idea at its core, namely, protecting fighters, but in doing so, it has only further complicated the framework. Sanctioning and regulatory decisions continue to be the purview of states, some of which cannot afford to provide simple things such as prefight drug testing; and while most athletic commissions pay ringside physicians without the involvement of the promotion, there are still a handful that cannot pay for medical services without the financial support of the promotion whose primary interest is often the production of the best fight card that will sell the most tickets.

And the "alphabet soup" of sanctioning bodies such as the WBA, IBF, WBC, ABC, IBC, and WBO will continue to complicate regulatory matters. While the push to protect fighters is strong, the constant addition of new sanctioning bodies and legislature favoring independent state decisions makes regulation even harder. With Duk-koo Kim looking down, it seems the cobra is still winning the round.

8

Tom Brady and Protecting the Quarterback

SOMETIMES WHEN THE SCALES FAVOR one group over another, trying to adjust the imbalance may end up tipping those unequal scales even farther. Such an example can be found in Mexico's answer to car pollution. When it comes to air quality, Mexico City is one of the world's most polluted cities. Stories have been told of birds literally dropping dead out of the sky from smog. On a measurable level, Mexico City has the worst air quality in the Western Hemisphere. Scientists have measured particulate levels that are three to four times higher than other major populated cities such as New York, Los Angeles, and São Paulo.

One of the major contributors to Mexico City's air pollution problem is car congestion. So in the 1980s, in an attempt to reduce the number of cars on the road, the Mexican government introduced a driving ban. The ban, called *Hoy No Circula*, restricted cars from driving on the roads one day a week based on the last digit of the license plate. Two numbers per workday were used. So, for example, if a license plate ended in a 1 or 2, that car would be banned from driving on Mondays. If it ended in 3 or 4, it would be banned on Tuesdays, and so on. If effective, the law would remove 20 percent of cars each workday (10 percent for each number 0 through 9 banned on that day) between the hours of 5 a.m. and 10 p.m.

In principle, it was a sound idea, but the people of Mexico City quickly found ways around the new law. One of the easiest and most direct ways to skirt the law was simply to buy another car with a new license plate. And rather than spend a ton of money on a fancy new car, all they had to do was buy a cheap gas-guzzler, which, in turn, would produce even more pollution. So, instead of forcing those who could afford a car to take public transportation, those who were already wealthy enough to own a car simply added another cheaper one to their collection. As a result, there is some evidence that the air pollution levels actually increased over the months after the driving ban was enacted. The poor, on the other hand, who could not afford their own car in the first place and already had to carpool, would need to find another carpool to use on those designated days.

In 2008, Mexico tried improving the car ban by adding in Saturdays, when fewer people were trying to get to work. Again, the day a car was banned (in this case two Saturdays of the month) was based on license plate numbers. And yet, following the updated ban, there still was no discernible effect on pollution. In a study published in the *Nature* journal's Scientific Reports, Lucas Davis from UC Berkeley's Haas School of Business analyzed hourly data from pollution-monitoring stations. He focused on the results following the expansion of the driving ban. Based on the data recorded for eight major pollutants, the program expansion had no discernible effect on Mexico City's pollution levels.

Davis further investigated how the bans affected public transportation ridership. The data showed no increases in subway, bus, or light rail ridership. The author concluded that since more people were not staying home and pollution levels were unchanged, then they were either carpooling or using services like taxis that didn't fall under the ban (Uber wasn't available yet). If the answer was that they were carpooling, then pollution levels would theoretically decrease, but only if they were all initially going to the same location. If carpools were adding new destinations to the same car, then the pollution level would continue to increase as the time and length of the drive increased.

Something Davis also brings up is the thought that someone wealthy enough could bribe their way to using a banned car, but due to enormous Mexican police presence and enforcement on these Saturdays, one would have to bribe a lot of people along the way at multiple spots. So, in the end, an attempt to make Mexico City's air quality healthier may have actually made things worse for the environment and for the poor, and those people fortunate enough to have money for a car simply found easier ways around the ban.

Another example where we see a direct effect of furthering inequality on those who might already need protection is found deep down in Mississippi, along the levees. The Mississippi River has a devastating flood history, most recently in both 2016 and 2017. But one of the worst in history happened in 2011, leading to over $3 billion dollars in damage to the area's agriculture and infrastructure. Flooding of the mighty Mississippi, however, is nothing new. It's been recorded for at least 150 years. In the 19th century, levees were instituted as a means of controlling the fluctuating water levels, but soon they became overwhelmed and resulted in more flooding. What became apparent pretty quickly was that if you tried to push the mighty river into a small, narrow channel, the water levels in the channel would just rise faster and the spillover would become even more powerful and devastating.

In response to a major flood in 1927, the Army Corps of Engineers designed a system of levees, dams, spillways, and channels to help control the overflow. Unfortunately, this has not stopped the problem and has led to its own resultant cycles of flooding and land loss that in turn necessitate further flood control and land restoration. While the variability of the river flooding is partly related to how hot or cold the oceans are, it's really the levee system that seems to be the main culprit. By protecting some parts of the city with levees, the floods are diverted to less protected neighborhoods. In a research letter to *Nature*, a large group of scientists hailing from across the United States and as far as the UK published their work on how the levees in Mississippi can actually amplify flood risk.

The authors concluded that human alterations to the Mississippi

River system combined with the effects of climate variability have "elevated the current flood hazard to levels that are unprecedented within the past five centuries." Ultimately, it's these floods that end up harming the agriculture and lands of different communities, so in a sort of Dr. Seuss-inspired levee war, each community raises the level of their levees, which only ends up hurting their neighbors on the unprotected side of the levees. This can go on back and forth. The end result is that when one group is protected by the levees, another group gets flooded, usually the poorer community. Here the cobra seems to ensure that when we try to make things safer and protect one group, we can end up making things worse for another already disenfranchised group.

TOM BRADY LINED UP BEHIND his snapper. The roar of the Super Bowl LIII crowd was deafening. It was the fourth quarter, and the New England Patriots were still tied, 3–3, with the Los Angeles Rams. Brady's team had just received the kick. They were starting with first-and-ten on the 31-yard line. He pointed to the defensive line, making a last-minute call adjustment, and then dropped back. First, he faked a handoff to a running back and then looked to his right. Tight end Rob Gronkowski pretended to block for a run play before sidestepping his defender. Gronkowski was one of Brady's favorite targets but had been quiet on offense for most of the game. Suddenly, shuffling to the side, "Gronk" got half a step ahead of his defender and motioned for the ball. Brady launched a lob pass to Gronkowski, who caught it midstride to give the Patriots a first down and a jolt of momentum. New England huddled up to discuss the next play as a chant of "Brady! Brady!" echoed throughout Mercedes-Benz Stadium in Atlanta.

The forty-one-year-old quarterback's team set back up on its own 49-yard line, more than half of the field separating them from the end zone. Reminiscent of childhood backyard football games everywhere, the storyline was set. The Vince Lombardi Super Bowl trophy was on the line with a tie game in the fourth quarter. Everyone knew Brady was no stranger to last-minute drives. Seven of his last eight Super Bowl appearances were decided in the final few minutes or in overtime.

He lined up behind the snapper for the next play. History was waiting for him downfield. It was no small feat for a man his age to be on the verge of leading his team to a record sixth Super Bowl victory. He had talent for sure and was one of the most reliable passers in the game, especially in do-or-die situations. His legacy was actively being crafted on that very field. Everyone's eyes were on the future and what was about to unfold. What most people didn't see that day was a past lurking behind him, a history filled with years of rule changes that helped ensure this general was still afforded adequate protection to lead his army into battle.

Few injuries are remembered as gruesomely as the day Lawrence Taylor tackled quarterback Joe Theismann. During a 1985 Monday Night Football game, Theismann, a quarterback for the Washington Redskins, handed off the football to his running back, who then tossed it right back to him in a trick play known as a "flea-flicker." As the passer looked downfield to throw the ball, one of the league's most-feared defensive players, Lawrence Taylor, leaped at Theismann from behind and started to bring him down. While the two of them were falling to the ground, Taylor's knee pushed Theismann's leg underneath the quarterback's own body. Gary Reasons, another large defensive player, also jumped onto the pack. Under the weight of three bodies, Theismann's own leg was bent backward and sandwiched between Taylor, Reasons, and himself. Once the mass of entangled bodies stopped moving, Taylor suddenly jumped to his feet and motioned for help from the sideline. He placed his hands on either side of his helmet in disbelief. What he saw was enough to shake him to his core. Theismann's leg was clearly and grossly deformed.

The Redskins quarterback was carted off the field and diagnosed with a "compound" or open fracture in which both the tibia and fibula broke about 1/3 up the leg from the ankle. The open nature means not only did the bones break, but they poked out of the skin, which carries an increased risk of infection. Theismann later told the *New York Times* in a 2005 interview that when he finally agreed to watch a video of the injury for the first time, "The pain was unbelievable, it snapped like a breadstick. It sounded like two muzzled gunshots off my left shoulder. Pow, pow!"

Dr. Charles Jackson, the Redskins' team physician, recalls evaluating the injury on the field. Theismann's knee was facing straight up, but his foot was flat on the ground. "So there is a tendency to want to straighten the leg out," he told the *Washingtonian*. "But if it's an open fracture, you can't do that because of the risk of infection. What you don't want to do is take a piece of dirt and pull it back up into the marrow of the bone. So we left his leg the way it was and splinted him right there on the spot." Theismann was then taken to the hospital, where the bones were surgically washed and straightened, the skin closed, and a cast placed. "Hollywood Joe," as he was called, never returned from the injury.

As a result of the freak play, the value of protecting a quarterback, especially on his "Blind Side," became a priority. The "Blind Side" of a right-handed quarterback trying to throw the ball is on his left side. When he turns his body to throw and points his left shoulder down the field, his back is to the left side and it becomes a wide-open target for a defender. The person standing between this defender and the quarterback is usually the left tackle. As a result, the left tackle has become one of the most significant positions on a sports roster.

The first person to bring this concept to the mainstream public was author Michael Lewis. He had been speaking to NFL front offices about the baseball-winning statistical strategy from his book *Moneyball*. During one meeting, Lewis was spending some time with the San Francisco 49ers organization when they showed him something that amazed even a best-selling sports author. The left tackle position, the player responsible for guarding the quarterback's "Blind Side," had gone from an overlooked positional player to the second-highest paid player on the team. Lewis recalled in 2015 to the *Washingtonian*, "I asked Bill Parcells, 'How did the left tackle get more and more valuable?' And he says, 'Lawrence Taylor'." Thanks to L.T., protecting the quarterback's left side morphed into one of the most important tasks on the football field.

Twenty years after Theismann's fateful game, the Cincinnati Bengals and Pittsburgh Steelers were facing off in the first round of the 2005 AFC playoffs. Quarterback Carson Palmer was in the midst of a promising season with high hopes for a Super Bowl appearance. In just the second play of the game, Palmer planted his back leg and let a pass fly. As soon as he let go of the ball, the opposing defender, Kimo von Oelhoffen, grabbed him by the leg and brought him to the ground. Palmer's back knee twisted and buckled. Von Oelhoffen described the pop in Palmer's knee like a gunshot going off next to his ear. An MRI revealed that Palmer had suffered a season-ending tear of his ACL and MCL. The early end to Palmer's run, or any quarterback's, was not something NFL owners liked to see. As a result, many of them felt they had to take action to protect their prized assets. Two months later, a new rule change was proposed during the 2006 NFL Owners' Meeting. The new rule required defenders to take every opportunity to avoid hitting a quarterback at or below the knees unless they were blocked directly into him.

Previously, a defender was only penalized if he hit a quarterback low during an unrestricted path to his target. With a free and direct line to the quarterback, it would be considered a low and dangerous blow to target the quarterback's legs. However, if the defender had been blocked in the process and gotten around said obstruction, he was no longer bound to the same rule and could lunge for the knees. With the so-called "Carson Palmer" rule, defenders had to take every opportunity to not hit the quarterback in the knees or shins, even if they were coming off a block and had a straight shot to the QB. If there was a chance to avoid the quarterback's legs, they had to take it. Ironically, though, von Oelhoffen's hit on Palmer likely would still not have been considered illegal under the rule change. The league had deemed he could not have avoided the hit.

There was some discussion among the coaches, owners, and representatives of the NFL's Competition Committee. Some defensive coordinators spoke up, saying they agreed with protecting the quarterback, but with the new rule, it would become "an officiating nightmare." It was important, they agreed, to keep the quarterback healthy. In fact, they wanted to keep all players healthy, but perhaps the rule went too far. A split arose between those who did not want to enter the possible quagmire of officiating a defensive player's intent and perhaps unfairly penalizing him versus potentially keeping a star franchise player healthy at all costs. At the session, nine votes would have been required to table the new rule change. It ended up passing with the first vote, 25–7. This level of protections seemed to suffice for two more years until the NFL lost an even bigger star just as a new season was dawning.

It was 2008. The year before, Tom Brady had led the New England Patriots to a perfect regular season. They had not lost a single game on their way to their Super Bowl. A championship win would have been the perfect end to a storybook season. They were easily the heavy favorites to win over the ragtag New York Giants. But in one of the biggest upsets in NFL history, the Patriots lost to the Giants, and Brady was robbed of his perfect ending. But now it was the first quarter of the first game of the new season. The reigning MVP was ready to avenge his team's Super Bowl loss. Brady took a snap and shuffled forward a few times ready to throw the ball downfield. At the same time, New England running back Sammy Morris blocked Kansas City Chief Bernard Pollard to the ground. As Brady went to release the ball, Pollard leaped low across the ground and seized Brady's lead left knee. Brady let out a scream and quickly knelt down. Unable to put much weight on his leg, the New England quarterback hobbled to the locker room with assistance. He would suffer the same fate as Carson Palmer—a torn ACL ended his season just as quickly as it began.

When arguably the best player in the league misses a season at the height of his career, the powers that be again take notice. The Patriots' owner summed it up this way to the *Boston Globe* in 2009: "I think the whole NFL suffers. . . . So whatever we can do to protect quarterbacks and to minimize the opportunity of them being taken out with a year-ending injury I would support." He continued, "It's not good for the league. What makes it special is special players. It's like going to see a great movie and the star isn't in the movie. It's the same principal." The NFL responded to the owners' renewed concerns by instituting a rule clarification of the previously labeled "Carson Palmer" rule. The clarification stated that defenders who were already on the ground were prohibited from lunging or diving at the quarterback's legs. Since this was not a new rule, but rather an adjustment to an already existing rule, it did not require the same voting by team owners.

Like the original rule before it, the change garnered mixed reactions. The controversy continued to lie in what was the true intention of the rule. In some circles, the rule change was nicknamed the "Brady Rule," because it was clearly formed in response to the high-profile Patriots player's injury. Prosafety advocates pointed to the rule as a form of injury risk reduction, whereas its opponents claimed its motivation was to overly protect franchise money-making players. Usually, these financially important players were quarterbacks like Tom Brady. It was seen as an openly biased decision. In doing so, the critics argued, it further inhibited the careers of less famous and less affluent defensive players. Since quarterbacks tended to be white, and defensive players black, some of the players viewed this as further racial inequality within the NFL. It also made on-the-field interpretation even murkier as to when a defensive player could get back into a play after being knocked to the ground.

The conversation of racial inequality is something that has surfaced several times in the NFL, most recently in regard to Colin Kaepernick's on-field protests. This important conversation even found its way back to *The Blind Side*. When the movie adaptation was released, there were some in the audience who felt it pushed a stereotypical racial inequality narrative. Some critics labeled it as just another "white-savior" story where a white family "saves" a black child from doom and poverty. On the other hand, there were some anecdotal reports that a few white families had been inspired by the movie and chose to adopt black children into their family. These were considered more positively spun stories and even relayed to Lewis himself. Michael Oher's adoptive mother from the book also used her new platform to promote adoption and foster care with a book and a TV show. So, if there truly was an uptick in foster care or adoption, it would be an uncanny connection between Joe Theismann's leg injury and a white family welcoming an African American child into their family thirty years later.

What has remained, statistically, is a disparate proportion of the racial makeup when it comes to positions on the football field. For a long time, African American football players were unofficially banned from playing the quarterback position. In today's era, we have seen examples of superstar black quarterbacks such as Cam Newton, Michael Vick, and Russell Wilson. But that was not always the case. For too long a time, black players were seen as lacking the intellect or leadership required to run the offense. It wasn't until 1988 that Doug Williams broke the football quarterback color barrier by becoming the first African American quarterback to lead his team to a Super Bowl championship.

One of the first African American players to really harness the reins as an NFL quarterback was Warren Moon. Moon was a top-rated player who was skipped over for the NFL draft out of college. Even if he had been drafted, it was assumed that he would have been forced to change positions. African American players were considered unqualified for the "thinking" positions, meaning those positions down the middle: quarterback, center, and inside linebacker. Moon chose instead to sign on with the Canadian Football League (CFL). As a black man in the "Great White North," Moon led his team, the Edmonton Eskimos, to a record five consecutive Grey Cup victories from 1978 to 1982. He also was the first quarterback to pass for 5,000 yards, achieving the feat in both 1982 and 1983. Then, in 1983, he was signed by the NFL's Houston Oilers. During an NFL career that spanned 16 years, he set more than 35 team franchise records (including the Tennessee Oilers and Tennessee Titans) that still stand today. Moon was also elected to the Canadian Football Hall of Fame in 2001 and has been ranked as number 5 in the top 50 CFL players of all time.

Despite the barrier breakers such as Moon and Williams, the quarterback is still a predominantly white position. Other positions that are also predominantly white are usually punters and kickers, which is likely because most of those players are converted from soccer, which in the United States is traditionally played in white neighborhoods. It's also worth pointing out, though, that white players who play traditionally black positions such as running back face stereotypes of their own. Every year, The Institute for Diversity and Ethics in Sports (TIDES) publishes statistics and report cards regarding gender and race in sports such as baseball, basketball, and football both at the collegiate and professional levels. In its most recent report for 2018, the NFL received an A- for its racial hiring practices, but only a C for its gender hiring practices. Data for the racial makeup of the NFL players were only available for 2016. Those data showed that 69.7 percent were African American and 27.4 percent were white. From available data in 2015, the biggest discrepancies on offense were found at quarterback (QB), running back (RB), wide receiver (WR), and center (C). The vast majority of QBs and centers were white and the vast majority of running backs and wide receivers were black. Further, when it comes to paying running backs, despite being some of the highest scorers on the team, these injury-prone position players earn on average less than kickers and punters.

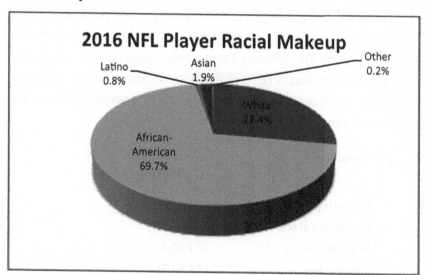

Data Source: TIDES 2018 NFL Racial and Gender Report Card: National Football League.

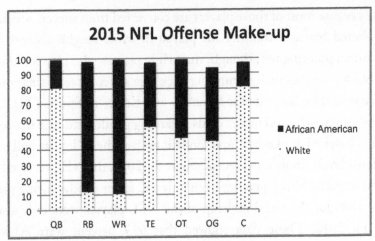

Source: TIDES 2015 NFL Racial and Gender Report Card:
National Football League.

There is even some research available as to which positions are at the greatest risk of being injured. Zachary Binney, PhD, MPH is an epidemiologist who spends his free time calculating statistics for the website Football Outsiders. He combed through the NFL's regular season weekly injury reports from 2007 to 2015. Using these data, he calculated injury rates by position per 1,000 athlete-exposures (AEs). One AE is defined as one player participating in one practice or game. What he found was that running backs topped the list for injury risk. The next highest are defensive backs, wide receivers, linebackers, and tight ends. Quarterbacks fall way down on the list at number eight out of the nine positions studied. Their injury risk is about 2.5 times less than that of running backs.

Position	Injury Rate per 1,000 AEs (Standard Error)
Running Back	20.7 (0.5)
Defensive Back	17.4 (0.3)
Wide Receiver	17.1 (0.4)
Linebacker	17.1 (0.3)
Tight End	16.9 (0.5)

Defensive Lineman	15.1 (0.3)
Offensive Lineman	12.8 (0.3)
Quarterback	8.6 (0.4)
Safety	4.4 (0.3)

NFL Injury Rates by Position per 1,000 Athlete-Exposures (AEs).
Data Source: Zachary Binney, PhD, MPH; FootballOutsiders.com.

From a brain trauma perspective, we can gather some data from a study published in the journal *Radiology* in 2017. It should be noted that both the NFL Players Association and the NFL Foundation helped fund the study. The researchers used MRIs to evaluate evidence of brain injury in 61 former collegiate and professional football players who were between the ages of 52 and 65 years old. What the group found was that career duration and player position affected white matter changes in the brain. Longer careers had greater risks, which wasn't that surprising. But what was interesting was that there was a difference in evidence of brain injury on MRI between "speed" and "nonspeed" positions. Speed players were considered to be positions such as running back, quarterback, or wide receiver, whereas nonspeed positions were either offensive or defensive linemen. Based on the data, it appeared linemen were at the greatest risk of developing white matter changes, especially in the front, where there might be more helmet-to-helmet contact while blocking.

Following the 2006 and 2009 rule changes, there was a measurable change in how teams played the game and how the quarterbacks performed. The total number of touchdowns thrown in the league during each season jumped significantly. In 2006, when Carson Palmer was hurt, the league threw a total of 648 TDs. In 2007, after the rule change, there were 720 TDs thrown. In 2009, when Tom Brady was hurt, the league threw 710 TDs. After the rule modification for 2010, there were 751 total TDs. In fact, if you look at the trend from 2000 to 2018, there is a general upward trend (as there has been since the beginning of the NFL), but most notably there are no seasons that have more touchdowns thrown than the one when the Brady rule was incorporated. There is clearly a level change starting after the Brady rule change in 2010. The only low point seemed to occur in 2017. But even this low sits above the highest total touchdown number from before the rule change.

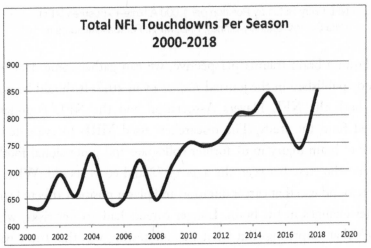

Data Source: ProFootballReference.com.

There is no doubt NFL owners know what defines their financial bottom line, and an investment in a quarterback is not something they want to lose money on. Healthier, well-protected quarterbacks equal more throwing touchdowns and better chances at winning Super Bowls. However, preventing the loss of a quarterback, or even protecting the quarterback so much that high-scoring passing TDs become the norm, may not actually be a good thing for the league. If we look at yearly trends for the NFL, more TDs and healthier QBs don't seem to translate into improved ratings. In fact, the opposite may be happening. If we look at NFL ratings by year, we see a general downward trend. The year Brady returned from his ACL surgery actually saw one of the biggest increases in NFL viewership ratings compared to the previous year. But then things start to decline. There was somewhat of an increase again from 2009 to 2010, but after 2010, NFL ratings hardly ever increased and, in most cases, declined.

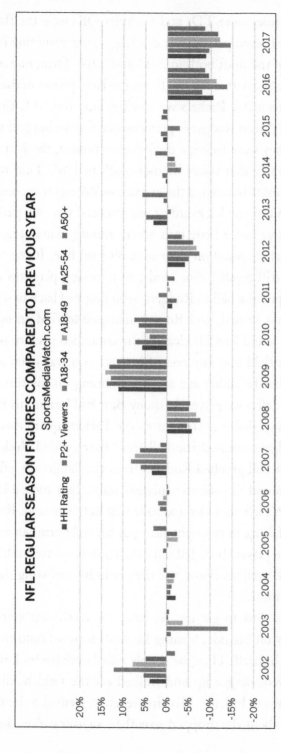

NFL REGULAR SEASON FIGURES COMPARED TO PREVIOUS YEAR

SportsMediaWatch.com

■ HH Rating ■ P2+ Viewers ■ A18-34 ■ A18-49 ■ A25-54 ■ A50+

Nielsen Ratings: Household Ratings (HH), People Ages Two and Up Viewership (P2+), Adults 18–34, Adults 18–49, and Adults 25–54.
Source: SportMediaWatch.com.

Still, for a while, more TDs and healthier QBs were the flavor of the day. The NFL even passed over drafting a single running back in the first round of the draft both in 2013 and 2014. Then, one Sunday in 2017, things took another big hit. It was the first quarter of the Week 6 game. The Green Bay Packers were riding atop the NFC division, and quarterback Aaron Rodgers's performance was an integral part of their success. They were facing a divisional opponent, the Minnesota Vikings, in a rivalry that traces its roots back to 1961. That was the year when Minnesota welcomed the expansion Vikings team next door to Wisconsin and in the backyard of the Packers. On this particular Sunday, there were just a little over seven minutes remaining in the quarter. The Packers stood on their own 39-yard line. It was second down and they still needed nine yards, so a passing play was called. The center snapped the ball to Rodgers, who dropped back to scan the field. The defense rushed, and Rogers managed to find an opening to his right. He found himself clear of the entangled pack of players. He looked downfield and saw one of his receivers was open and let the ball fly. What he didn't see as he was lining up his throw was that Minnesota defensive player Anthony Barr had beaten his blocker and had an unimpeded line straight to the Packers quarterback. No sooner had Rodgers released the ball than Barr tackled Rodgers to the ground. Barr had grabbed Rodgers from the dangerous left blind side, his hand around the offensive player's waist. Barr tucked his helmet into Rodgers's left shoulder and rode him to the ground. Rodgers, feeling himself falling to the right side, put his right arm out to brace himself. The two players both fell onto the Packers quarterback's right arm. They rolled over his elbow and then onto his throwing shoulder from the momentum.

Rodgers was slow to get up. At first, the tenth-year starter for the team just lay on his side, leaning his head forward onto the field trying to gather himself. Then, he simply rolled onto his back in pain. Once help arrived, he got up and walked off the field holding his arm straight down at his side. His first reaction seemed to be that he was more upset about the dropped pass than anything else. But after a few more minutes, his shoulder became a greater concern, and he was carted off the field and into the locker room. X-rays revealed a displaced clavicle, or collarbone, fracture that would require surgical stabilization with two plates and screws. It was a devastating blow to the Packers, robbing them of their leader for all but one game during the rest of the season.

In response to Rodgers's injury, members of the NFL's Competition Committee felt a change needed to be made regarding how much of a defender's body weight could be used while driving a quarterback to the ground. The initial wording of the rule had been crafted back in 1995. It stated that "When tackling a passer during or just after throwing a pass, a defensive player is prohibited from unnecessarily and violently throwing him down and landing on top of him with all or most of the defender's weight." Following the committee's conference, this statement was amended. For the upcoming 2018 season, the rule would be interpreted as "a defensive player is prohibited from unnecessarily and violently throwing him down OR [emphasis added by author] landing on top of him with all or most of the defender's weight." As a result, if a defensive player landed on top of a passing quarterback with most of his weight, the referee would be obligated to penalize him for roughing the passer—an infraction that carried a 15-yard penalty and automatic first down for the offense.

By the third week of the 2018 season, media, players, fans, and even former officials were up in arms. In the 2017 season, the league saw just 16 roughing the passer penalties through Week 3. That number more than doubled to 34 in the same time frame of 2018. Also in that same third week, Dolphins defensive end William Hayes had sped toward Raiders quarterback Derek Carr in the Miami-Oakland game. During the sack, Hayes seemed to recognize the new ruling and attempted to sprawl onto the field without putting all of his body weight onto Oakland's franchise offensive player. As a result of the awkward movement to protect the quarterback, Hayes ended up tearing his own ACL. In the attempt to avoid a penalty from a rule designed to protect the quarterback, the defensive end suffered his own significant knee injury.

Critics pounced on this as a perfect illustration of the absurdity of the new rule enforcement. How, they asked, is a 250-to-300-pound defensive player supposed to run at a quarterback, begin to tackle him, and then somehow in midair change his body's trajectory so that he doesn't land on top of the quarterback? Even Joe Theismann, whose leg injury sparked the era of quarterback protections, felt the NFL had begun to protect quarterbacks too much. In an interview with Stuart Varney, he stated, "I think the rule has crossed the line when it comes to safety. I am all for protecting the quarterback—you can barely touch them anymore but how do you stop someone who is coming after the quarterback and asking them in an instant to change what their body is going to do?" It certainly seems like an impossible feat for the defender to perform. Proponents of the rules again point to quarterback safety and financial bottom lines. After all, there were likely many more Derrick Carr jerseys in the stadium that day than William Hayes jerseys. Quarterbacks are an important position and a big financial investment for an NFL team. But they say defense wins championships. So who is protecting the defensive players? Are the NFL scales, already favoring quarterbacks over defensive players, being tilted farther by the cobra snake's unintended consequences? One thing we do see is that the pass rusher is now one of the highest-paid players on the team simply because his job is to try and get to the quarterback and prevent him from throwing. And yet, the offensive machine keeps rolling on, at least for the passers and receivers. The 2018 season was a record-setting year of touchdowns. The 1,371 touchdowns scored in the regular season were the most for a single season in the 99-year history of the league. Quarterbacks were throwing more touchdown passes than ever. Tom Brady reached the record for most combined touchdown passes in the regular season and post-season. And for the first time ever, both of the teams in a single game scored 50 or more points.

So, when Tom Brady dropped back to throw the ball in the fourth quarter of Super Bowl LIII, it was considered largely an unexciting game, mostly due to the lack of offense. The defense was doing its job and keeping the football out of the end zone. At 41, Brady was the oldest quarterback ever in a Super Bowl, and nearly one of the oldest Super Bowl players ever. The title of oldest player is actually held by kicker Matt Stover, who was 42 years old when he played in Super Bowl XLIV. Protected by his offensive line, and perhaps the rulebook, Brady did what he was known for. He found an open receiver downfield with only minutes left in the game. The aged veteran then marshaled his team to a game-winning touchdown and a record sixth Super Bowl victory. Yet, we must wonder, if the NFL hadn't made protecting the quarterback a priority with each rule change, would Tom Brady at his age still be standing at the helm?

9

Tiger's Back

IT WAS 1927 IN WASHINGTON, DC, and the city was preparing for another invasion. Just a few nights prior, an employee in the District Building had accidentally left a window open, and a swarm of the invaders had made their way inside. They were forced out the next day, but everyone knew they would be back. So this time, the city erected four massive floodlights on the outside of the federal building. Hopefully, the massive bright spotlights would scare the trespassers away. Previous efforts at repelling the dark marauders had failed. Two years earlier, the fire department had tried spraying them with powerful hoses, only to find out most had left their encampment under darkness the night before. The few who were left, according to the *Washington Post*, "disappeared down Pennsylvania Avenue uttering what sounded surprisingly like a horse laugh." Even the White House and US Capitol were on alert. The columns around the Capitol were wrapped with electrified wire, and the president's own home had speakers installed to emit what sounded like owl calls to drive the would-be intruders away.

The clue to the start of this conflict, it was said, could be traced back as far as Shakespeare—specifically to *Henry IV* Part I. Act I, Scene 3. The scene in question took place inside London's royal palace. In anger, King Henry IV had summoned Sir Henry Percy to Windsor Castle. Harry Hotspur, as the eldest son of Northumberland was called, was accompanied by his father, the Earl of Northumberland, and his uncle, the Earl of Worcester. The British ruler demanded to know why Hotspur had failed to hand over the prisoners he captured in Scotland.

Hotspur tells the king that he will only hand over the prisoners if the crown pays a ransom to release his captured brother-in-law, Mortimer. Henry refuses, calling Mortimer a traitor. The king then storms out, leaving the Northumberland crew to plan their next move. Hotspur, clearly enraged, vows to sneak upon the king while he is sleeping and yell "Mortimer" in his ear. He then amends the plan. He has a far more devious idea. He will find a starling and teach it to say, "Mortimer." It will haunt Henry by repeating the name over and over again, perpetually enraging the king. Throughout his wide volume of work, this is the one and only time Shakespeare mentions the invasive bird that can mimic the human voice. Yet, that mere mention of a starling would lead to another act of unfolding unforeseen consequences 300 years later.

The next act in this tale takes place on the cold, winter morning of March 6, 1890. Sleet is blanketing Central Park. On the stage, a New York pharmaceutical manufacturer named Eugene Schieffelin steps into history's spotlight. Schieffelin is both a huge fan of Shakespeare and of birds. Naturally, he concocts a scheme to combine his two loves. He will introduce every type of bird mentioned in Shakespeare's plays into North America. It was a simple problem: these birds were only found in Europe. So he had a simple fix: he would release them in Central Park. Other groups had failed with the introduction of nightingales and skylarks, but where they failed, he and his 60 starlings would succeed. Having made the long journey from Schieffelin's country house to the heart of New York City in cages, the birds immediately took to the sky upon their release. They fought the thick snow and heavy wind before finding shelter under the overhanging roof of the nearby American Museum of Natural History.

Shattering the expectations of those who knew of their impending release, the birds would not only survive that frigid night, they would survive the entire winter and beyond. Under the watchful eye of carved eagles, they would breed amongst the Victorian Gothic towers, and their numbers would grow. Soon, the original flock of 60 birds would number over 100 million. They would reach as far as Washington, DC, in the 1920s. By the 1990s, the avian army would double its ranks to nearly 200 million with outposts stretching from Alaska to Mexico. And with the expansion came the destruction. Each year, the birds would cause hundreds of millions of dollars in damage. Their droppings are corrosive, and their large nests can carry fungus and mites. They drive away native species. In 2008, US government agents attempted to retaliate by poisoning, shooting, and trapping nearly 2 million starlings, and yet they made no dent in the starling expansion.

Perhaps the most devastating effect of the starlings has been within the aviation industry. These black birds fly in large, moving swarms across the sky. They mimic a large ink puddle stretching and collapsing like a lava lamp in the sky—the shape of which seamlessly transitions from one random Rorschach pattern to the next. When they come across air traffic, they form large clouds that can suddenly get sucked up into airplane engines. The most deadly bird-strike crash in US history occurred in 1960, when an Eastern Air Lines plane crashed shortly after taking off from Boston. The plane had run into a flock of starlings immediately after takeoff. The birds were sucked into three of its four engines. The entire windshield was covered in black. Stalling in midair, the plane spiraled downward and plunged into Boston Harbor, killing 62 of the 72 people on board. The entire tragedy seemed to take less than a minute to unfold.

With what seemed like a simple fix to a problem, Eugene Schieffelin set into motion a series of events that led to a perpetuation of problems. Releasing just 60 birds led to millions of dollars in damage and the loss of several lives. If we are not careful, a plan for a quick fix may shield our attention from appreciating potential consequences. With a seemingly innocuous act, we might be setting the stage for the cobra to introduce a new tragic tale. Sometimes it's not a starling who gets the quick fix, but rather a Tiger.

On May 29, 2017, at 2:03 a.m., Florida police officer Matthew Palladino pulled up to examine what appeared to be a motor vehicle crash. It was Memorial Day, so patrol units were on the lookout for drunk drivers. He radioed in what he saw. There was a black Mercedes parked in the right-hand traffic lane of Military Trail. It was a long, dark road, but he could see the stopped car still had its brake lights on. The red taillights illuminated the back of the car and the license plate. With the aid of the light from the car's right-hand turn blinker flashing in the darkness, he scanned the pavement in front of the vehicle. Slowly, with his flashlight in hand, the officer approached the car. It was still running. The tires were flat. Inside, he saw a black male with his seat belt on dressed in black athletic shorts and a white athletic shirt. His shoes were untied. He was slumped over the wheel, asleep.

The officer approached the driver and stirred him awake. His flashlight illuminated the face of the black male. For a split second, he had an uncanny resemblance to one of the town's famous residents. Another car pulled up, and Officer Palladino was soon joined by other officers. Officer Fandrey first spoke with the officers on the scene, was handed a driver's license, and then himself approached the vehicle. Using the flashlight in his other hand, he looked down at the card he was holding. The face he saw matched the picture on the license, but he knew he didn't need the card to identify the man who was asleep at the wheel. This man was Tiger Woods. The driver's license had his picture and his real name, Eldrick Tiger Woods, next to it. A positive ID was made. He began to speak to the driver, who had slow, slurred speech. He wasn't sure exactly where he was. He kept closing his eyes trying to doze off. At first, he thought he was heading back from golfing in Los Angeles. Then he realized he might have been headed to his house in Hobe Sound—but his car was facing the wrong direction. Woods volunteered that he recently had several surgeries and was taking several prescription medications.

The police officers helped him out of the vehicle. One of the officers tried to perform some roadside tests on the famous golfer. Using a flashlight, he could not get Woods's pupils to react and couldn't get him to follow the light with his eyes. The golfer was unable to walk along a line, stand on one foot, or move his fingers to his nose. Woods was then asked to close his eyes, tilt his head back, and say the alphabet backward without singing it. According to the police's records, when they asked Woods if he understood what was being requested, Woods replied he was asked to sing the national anthem backward. The instructions were then repeated, and the pro golfer got himself ready to speak but then turned and tried to wander off. He was steadied by the officers. After a few more minutes, he successfully completed the alphabet, at which point his hands were placed behind his back and handcuffed. Tiger Woods was under arrest.

Soon after, a breathalyzer test was performed and read a 0.00 level of alcohol content. It appeared he hadn't been drinking. His blood, however, would tell a different story. Tests came back positive for THC (the active ingredient in marijuana), Ambien (a sleep drug), Xanax (a drug for anxiety and depression), and two prescription painkillers, Vicodin and the even stronger Dilaudid. Woods would later blame his intoxicated state and the car crash on mixing medications to treat back pain and insomnia. That same back pain up until that point had been the greatest limiting factor in his professional career.

Few athletes have achieved such greatness that their name alone speaks of their dominance. Michael Jordan bears this crown in basketball. Muhammad Ali demands the same awe for boxing. Tiger Woods has wears the mantle for golf. His dominance on the golf course would begin with his drive, where a violent rotational explosion would send the ball careening toward its destination. An integral part of his game and who he was, this same powerful motion also wreaked havoc on his body. It caused his back to break down. Tiger had managed comebacks from neck pain, Achilles tendon injuries, and even an ACL rupture in his knee. He overcame those injuries, and until his back began to bother him, Tiger was the most dominant player on the PGA Tour. He was ranked number one in the world all but four years within the 16-year span of 1998 to 2013. Of those four years, during three of them he was ranked number two or three. His only hiccup was in 2011, when he injured his knee MCL and his Achilles tendon. Even when he underwent ACL reconstruction surgery in 2008, he still ended the year ranked number one.

The world first took notice of Tiger's back in August 2013. On the 13th hole at Liberty National, he lined up for his second shot in the fairway as the wind began to pick up. He let the club fly, and the ball sailed into the air. As the crowd watched, the ball veered significantly to the left and landed in a swamp 40 to 50 yards from the green. Tiger, meanwhile, dropped to his hands and knees grimacing in pain. He slowly got up and finished the round, but his back, and legacy, was never the same. On March 2, 2014, Tiger was warming up for Sunday's final round of the Honda Classic. He was ranked at the top of the golf world. He had just finished off his best round of the year on Saturday shooting a 5-under-par 65. This was a welcome change, because he admittedly hadn't had a good start to the year. He began 2014 by missing the cut in the Farmers Insurance Open at Torrey Pines, a tournament he had already won eight times before. Then, the following week, he finished in a tie for 41st in the Dubai Desert Classic. He was feeling a turn-around, though. He was going to get out of his slump.

Suddenly, he began to feel a tightening in his back. He tried to shake it, but the sharp, shooting pain kept coming back. He managed the best he could for the day but was falling far behind on the leaderboard. On the 9th hole, he started to rub his back and went over to talk to his girlfriend, skier Lindsey Vonn. He tried some stretches on the 11th hole, but the pain remained. The mighty golfer managed a par on the 13th hole, but once the ball clinked into the cup, he walked over to his playing partner, shook his hand, and turned in his scorecard. He just kept walking and exited the course. He was unable to return. Instead, he grabbed the hand of his daughter and hopped in a van to the parking lot, where he met up with Vonn, his caddie, and his son, who were all waiting for him.

Tiger would return to the golf course a week later and muscle through his back pain to finish the Cadillac Championship outside of Miami in Doral, Florida, but as anyone watching could tell, the back pain became too much for him to bear. Tiger announced he wouldn't play the upcoming Arnold Palmer Invitational due to continued back pain. At one point, he was practicing on a minicourse, and a small swing made him feel like he had been shot, sending him falling to the ground. He actually lay helplessly on the ground until his daughter found him. On April 1, 2014, Woods announced he would miss the Masters after undergoing a microdiscectomy the day before in Utah.

A microdiscectomy is performed when the gelatinous disc that sits between two spinal bones (vertebrae) has been injured and part of the disc bulges out, hitting a nerve. Now, most orthopedic and spine surgeons will tell you that simply having a disc bulge isn't a problem. In fact, many people have disc bulges but most don't bulge out far enough to pinch a nerve. However, if a nerve does get pinched, the pain can be considerable and usually shoots down the same path the nerve follows from the back to the legs. Removing part of the disc can take the pressure off of the nerve, but there is no guarantee that the disc bulge won't return. About 5 to 7 percent of patients will need a revision lumbar discectomy at some point. Woods would return to golf after his first surgery but would go on to miss the cut in three of the four major tournaments of 2015. He would undergo a second microdiscectomy in September of that year to remove another disc fragment that was pinching his lumbar nerve. Despite his doctor claiming the surgery was a complete success, persistent back pain led Tiger to a third surgery just one month later. The great golfer would retreat from the public spotlight to deal with chronic back pain and insomnia.

Woods would return to golf, but in 2016, he withdrew from play once again, this time before the second round of the Dubai Desert Classic, citing back spasms. Someone who saw him at a luncheon in Beverly Hills around that time thought he looked like a ninety-year old man shuffling around. He even had to walk up the stairs backward. And he had the glassy eyes of someone who may have been overmedicated. Eventually, Tiger consigned himself to undergoing a fourth back surgery. In this case, Woods underwent a fusion of the L5-S1 vertebrae. This is where the lowest lumbar bone (L5) meets the top of the first sacral bone (S1). In a fusion procedure, the disc between the two bones is completely removed so it can no longer bulge (if any of it is even left after multiple microdiscectomies), and the bones above and below the disc are fused together. In Woods's case, the idea was to relieve pain, since there would no longer be any motion or disc bulging at the affected spine level. The downside would be he would lose some motion at the fused spot. Fortunately for Woods, there is less motion at L5-S1 than there is elsewhere, especially compared to the thoracic spine (rib cage). In fact, the whole lumbar (lower back) spine accounts for only about 10 degrees of rotation versus about 45 degrees for the thoracic spine. Within the lumbar spine, the L5-S1 accounts for only about 1 to 2 degrees, but when it comes to physics, energy, and professional players, those 1 to 2 degrees can make a difference. Furthermore, once a level is fused, the adjacent levels see increased stress and can begin to break down (if not already wearing away in Woods's back). Tiger underwent the spinal fusion procedure on April 20, 2017.

As for rehabbing his back, Tiger needed to readjust his swing and to look for less power generation. Phil Mickelson, another top-level golfer, told the *New York Times* in 2016, "You can play golf for a lifetime and injury-free if you swing the club like Bobby Jones did and like Ernest Jones used to teach, where it's a swinging motion rather than a violent movement. A lot of the young guys continue to get hurt as they create this violent connected movement." Tiger himself admitted that his back pain was a different foe. With his previous injuries, the pain would occur after he hit the ball. So, even though it would hurt, the ball was already on its way to the intended target. With the back pain, it affected what he could do or how he could swing. That is something he needed to deal with in a different way, and that caused him to have to learn new strategies to overcome it.

Following his arrest in May, one month after his spinal fusion surgery, Tiger rented out the entire male inpatient unit of the Jupiter Medical Center hospital and focused on rehabbing from his substance abuse. Then in July 2017, he announced he had completed his intensive drug treatment. In August, he pleaded guilty to driving under the influence, and in December he finally got back out to the golf course. That month, Tiger was ranked as low as 1,119th in the world. But as of the time this chapter was written in early 2019, he has risen to the rank of 12th. He has also added a new chapter in his book. In April 2019, Tiger Woods became the second-oldest person ever to win the Masters Tournament at the age of 43. Tiger first won the Masters at age 21, less than a year after turning pro, and then won it again in 2001, 2002, and 2005. It was also the first time on a major championship golf course, and perhaps in his life, that Tiger had to come from behind to win. But as with his golf swing, his back is only one link in the chain of unintended consequence. For without his chronic back pain and surgeries, he may not have become dependent on prescription painkillers.

The use of opioids after surgery and subsequent addiction has been labeled a national "crisis." There is no doubt that there is an epidemic of opioid abuse across the country, and some of those stories can be traced back to narcotic pain medication use after surgery. Tiger's first major surgery was in 2008 to reconstruct his ACL. He had actually played without his ACL for some time. In fact, his doctors had told him it was almost completely torn after they examined it during his knee arthroscopy in 2002. And then in 2007, the remaining fibers completely tore, leaving him without an important stabilizing ligament in his knee. The ACL is a thick rope-like structure that's important for cutting, pivoting, and changing directions. Basically, whenever you plant your foot and turn quickly, without your ACL, your thigh bone (femur) and shin bone (tibia) won't stay together, and your knee will buckle and potentially tear something else inside your knee.

Without a stable ACL, Tiger's knee developed stress fractures within the bone. The ACL doesn't grow back on its own, so in order to stabilize his knee, Tiger needed an ACL reconstruction. His ACL surgery occurred on June 24, 2008. He likely was given some amount of prescription pain medication, because, for most people, this can be a painful surgery from which to recover. Up until that point, however, Tiger was no stranger to pain medication. It's not unheard of for elite athletes to turn to pain medication to get through a competition. He was first known to use pain medication in 2002, and by 2008, he was using Vicodin to get through the Masters tournament. The pain was nothing that some drugs couldn't get him through, he told his coach at the time.

The idea of getting an athlete through a game or tournament, or even the playoffs, is actually part of the "art" of treating the high-level athlete. What a sports medicine doctor prescribes is often dictated by whether an athlete is "in-season" or "out-of-season." An in-season athlete may have a lot riding on a particular game or perhaps it's the do-or-die playoffs and if they don't play, their team, or they, may never play again. In that case, a team doctor may try to get an athlete through a particular event as long as it's not against the standard of care to do so. There may be risks involved, but the athlete should be aware of them and make an educated decision. Then, when the season is over, more invasive or more impactful treatment may occur. For ACL surgery, however, there really is no good time. It's basically a season-ending injury that requires at least 6, and more likely 8 to 12 months of postoperative rehabilitation.

From an athletic and functional standpoint, Tiger recovered from his surgery. He was able to jog again, something he had been doing his entire career. Jogging allowed him to reach a greater level of fitness than his opponents. Like the movie character Rocky, Tiger would jog before "the fight" on the links. It seemed like he was back on track, but then on November 27, 2009, a new storyline emerged. That night, Tiger got into an argument with his then-wife over his infidelity. The model and mother of his children chased him out of the house with a golf club. Tiger attempted to drive off but ended up in the hospital. His SUV hit a fire hydrant, sending his car careening into a tree. The force of the impact knocked him unconscious. He also suffered several cuts on his face, whose origins were a point of dispute. Paramedics arrived on the scene and rushed Tiger to the hospital. His wife handed the paramedics two bottle of pills Tiger used. He had been using Ambien and Vicodin that night. Tiger would survive that night, but the next time Ambien and Vicodin would rear their heads would be when he was found asleep at the wheel of another car crash in 2017.

1998	1
1999	1
2000	1
2001	1
2002	1
2003	1
2004	1
2005	1
2006	1
2007	1
2008	1
2009	1
2010	2
2011	23
2012	3
2013	1
2014	32
2015	416
2016	652
2017	656
2018	13

Tiger Woods's PGA Rankings by Year. Source: Official World Golf Rankings, owgr.com.

To the average person, golf isn't a professional sport usually associated with chronic pain and injuries, whereas it's rather easy for someone to picture a nagging football injury, for example. Chronic injuries are the name of the game when money and careers are involved at the highest level of sports.

Unfortunately, in an unintended consequence of treating their injuries, many of these players end up abusing pain medications to do what they believe is their job—to go out and play even if it hurts. In a study published in July 2011, researchers from the Department of Psychiatry at Washington University School of Medicine in St. Louis teamed up with members of ESPN and contacted 644 retired NFL players. When all was said and done, their efforts snagged about 53 percent of the retired players to answer the survey.

In what are sobering statistics, over half (55 percent) of the players surveyed reported suffering a career-ending injury, and the average number of concussions they felt they had suffered was a staggering nine. In regard to pain medicine abuse, nearly one-third (29.4 percent) of the surveyed players felt that their teammates misused prescription opioids. And of the 52 percent of surveyed players who themselves had used opioids during their career, only 37 percent obtained their opioids exclusively from a doctor. A smaller percentage (12 percent) got them exclusively from a nonmedical source. The remaining majority (51 percent) of those who used opioids reported that the source of their prescription opioids was a combination of both doctors and other sources. These illicit sources included such people as their teammates, coaches, athletic trainers, and family members.

In a later study, researchers from the University of Florida sought to determine what led to opioid abuse after retirement from the NFL. This group included Linda Cottler, who was the lead author on the first NFL opioid study and specialized in research on the consequences of addiction. Her group also surveyed retired NFL players and found that about 12 percent admitted to using opioids without a prescription in the 30 days before the interview. When the researchers tried to find any risk factors for using opioids after retirement, they found two significant ones. The first was that they had used prescription opioids to "function" while in the NFL. The second was that they used the opioids while playing to "reduce stress and anxiety."

Stress and anxiety are no strangers to professional sports, especially in golf. World-championship-caliber golfers can suddenly be stricken by the dreaded "yips." The yips are an actual condition where a golfer can no longer smoothly putt or hit the ball. Instead, without warning, an unconscious jerky movement sends the ball travelling past or away from the intended target. It also certainly doesn't help when millions of dollars in purse money are on the line. With so much at stake at the professional level, it's only natural that PGA golfers would turn to medication to give them an advantage in combating nerves and anxiety. Public speakers, musicians, and other professionals have long turned to a medication that can slow the heart rate down to help them perform. These medications are known as beta-blockers, and up until 2008, they were perfectly legal to take while out on the links.

In 2012, legendary golfer Greg Norman remarked to the *New York Times*, "In my day, lots of guys were on beta blockers. It wasn't openly acknowledged, but it was obvious to the rest of us. A guy's personality would change. In practice rounds or friendly matches, we'd see the real guy under stress. Then in competition, he was like a different, calmer person." Norman would go on to say, "Those guys were trying to take the nerves out of the game. But nerves are very much a part of the game." In 2008, the same year Tiger played through both an ACL tear and stress fractures of his knee, the PGA instituted drug testing and began to ban certain medications such as beta-blockers. The guidelines were set up similar to but not exactly like the list compiled by the World Anti-Doping Association (WADA). That same year was also pivotal in the conversation surrounding performance-enhancing drugs. Tiger had been linked to Anthony Galea, a Canadian doctor who would later have his license suspended for providing elite athletes with the banned performance-enhancing drug Human Growth Hormone (HGH). Tiger's reason for the Canadian doctor's house calls was attributed to the use of Platelet Rich Plasma, or PRP, which is a procedure that happens in orthopedic offices across the globe. In the procedure, a patient's own blood is spun in a centrifuge until the layer with the platelets is isolated. Accompanying the platelets are signaling factors that can help promote healing. By injecting that layer, it's thought that a healing-friendly environment can be created.

Overall, results of studies with PRP are mixed. There seems to be some promise, but there still needs to be a fine-tuning of exactly which concentration of the healing factors should be used for the best effect and where the PRP is injected. When the news story broke, Tiger said Galea was simply helping him recover from his 2008 injuries and surgery. He had heard about Galea from Alex Rodriguez, who himself was recovering from a hip injury. Still, despite Tiger pointing to the PRP as the sole treatment provided by Galea, about one-quarter of PGA players still thought Tiger had at some point used performance-enhancing drugs. Recently, in 2019, a new book came out that has reignited the debate. In their book *Tiger Woods*, Jeff Benedict and Armen Keteyian report that one of their sources confirmed Tiger did receive HGH treatment during his recovery from his 2008 surgery, but it may have been done without his knowledge. Further, the level of HGH might have purposely been kept low to avoid detection. In response to this accusation, one of Tiger's doctors signed a statement specifically for the authors refuting this. Nevertheless, when the PGA announced its new testing policy in 2008, Tiger had his blood drawn and tested. He told his coach it was a precautionary measure due to the supplements he was taking.

Rumblings of potential PED abuse in the PGA, however, was not reason enough for many of the golfers on the tour to react well to newfound testing and oversight. Golf was generally considered a gentleman's game played under the code of honesty and self-policing. Penalties on the course were, after all, self-determined. In a statement to the Associated Press, Ryder Cup captain Paul Azinger expressed his dissatisfaction with having to perform a urine collection in front of a collector whose job was not only to make sure he urinated in a cup, but also to examine his exposed torso to make sure there were no false urine samples taped to his side. Another player, Frank Lickliter, told reporters that if anyone came to his house to collect the urine sample, as the policy allowed, they would be leaving with a bullet in their behind. Under the new rules, if a player was found in violation of the drug policy, it was up to the PGA's discretion to determine the punishment and also if the player and drug would be publicly identified. To many on the outside looking in, the PGA's drug-testing policy was deeply flawed. According to the policy, if a player was actually tested and a banned substance was detected, it was up to the commissioner to determine if the player would be suspended. If, for political or other reasons, the commissioner decided the player would get a pass, then no one outside the PGA walls would be notified of the failed drug test. The PGA protocol also couldn't test for HGH, simply because the drug wasn't detectable in urine. In an interview with Golf.com, WADA's own Director General David Howman said of the PGA testing program, "It's an invitation to break the rules."

One of the reasons Andy Levinson, the Tour's vice president for tournament administration and antidoping, said the PGA resisted blood-testing players was a concern that drawing a player's blood might affect his or her performance. Some players were still willing to provide blood samples, but not around tournament time, fearful that a needle poking their arms might affect their playing. They would allow themselves to be tested outside of competition, which was actually already in the new policy, but many top-level players admitted they were never tested outside of tournament venues. One of these players was Tiger Woods. The whole sentiment was simply summed up by Rory McIlroy, who was ranked number one in the world in both 2012 and 2014: "I could use HGH and get away with it."

This would all change in early 2017, three weeks almost to the day after Tiger crashed his car under the influence of a cocktail of pain and anxiety medications. On June 20, 2017, the PGA announced that for its next golf season, it would bring its drug-testing policies into closer alignment with the WADA policies. As such, the golf organization would add blood testing that could detect the other performance-enhancing drugs that urine could not, including HGH. In addition, it would release the names of drug policy violators as well as the name of the substance detected in the failed drug test. WADA's annual list of prohibited substances is harmonized across all sports. In order for a substance to be considered for inclusion on the list, it must meet two of the following three criteria: 1) It has the potential to enhance sport performance; 2) It represents a health risk to the athletes; and/or 3) It violates the spirit of sport. Two of the five drugs in Tiger's blood the night he crashed his car would fall under the new 2018 ban, namely, the THC from marijuana and the hydromorphone (Dilaudid). These are currently listed in the sections CANNABINOIDS and NARCOTICS, which follow each other on page 27 of the 2017–2018 USGA Anti-Doping Manual. The other major drug that Tiger had taken, Xanax, would still be legal under the Approved Anti-Anxiety medications section. That news was certainly welcome to golfer Charlie Beljan.

Charlie was a 28-year-old golfer who was heading into the second round of the PGA Children's Miracle Network Hospitals Classic when suddenly he felt as if his world were collapsing around him. He couldn't catch his breath, and he was overcome by a feeling of dread. His heart was racing. And yet, he still continued to play. Charlie had experienced a panic attack before, and this felt like another one. After finishing the round, he spent the night at a nearby hospital undergoing a series of tests, all of which came back negative. So, with the tournament on the line, Charlie returned to the course the next day for the final round. What followed can only be described as bizarre when the scene unfolded. The announcers discussed on the air how Charlie was actively having shortness of breath and an elevated heart rate. The tournament doctors had seen and examined him and cleared him to play. Alternating between sitting in the grass and stopping to catch his breath, with a medical crew following him around in a van, Charlie actually managed not only to finish, but also to win the tournament. He later consulted with several doctors, who all recommended medication for his anxiety and panic attacks. Certain medications for his symptoms, such as the beta-blockers Greg Norman described, were no longer legal on the PGA tour. Xanax, however, was still legal under WADA rules. Using the approved medication to control his anxiety, Charlie would avoid an early retirement and go on to compete in many other tournaments.

If you recall from the NFL Players Association study, the second risk factor for long-time opioid abuse was to "reduce stress and anxiety." What's interesting is that there are actually scientific studies on the connection between anxiety and the aforementioned "yips." *New Yorker* contributor David Owen actually wrote a whole article on this very topic in 2014. Ironically, the inspiration for his story was playing a round of golf with Hank Haney, who was none other than Tiger Woods's coach at the time. (For the record, Haney will tell you he broke up with Tiger.) Haney had a very odd way of swinging. He would swing the club like a baseball bat and then almost without stopping or looking down, take another swing to hit the ball. His swing technique was not random, but rather crafted in response to the development of an involuntary disruptive movement of his hand and wrists, i.e., the "yips." Among other adjustments, Haney also noticed if he didn't focus his attention too much on the ball at his feet, and instead looked at the brim of his hat, he actually hit the ball better.

In the article, Owen, who is also a contributing editor at *Golf Digest*, interviews several sports psychologists and scientists who actually studied the yips. These scientists were able to show the yips were not a myth, but an actual condition by identifying involuntary muscle contractions on EMG. First developed by detecting signals that could make severed frog legs kick and dance, EMG, or electromyography, is the study of electrical signals of cells within the muscles by using very fine electrodes. With the use of EMG, a group of these researchers initiated a study of putting to catch the mythical yips. With objective data, they were able to record several of the subjects displaying involuntary and uncoordinated muscle contractions of both the wrist flexors and wrist extensors at the same time, something that could easily throw a golf putt or swing off. Sometimes the golfers themselves weren't even aware of it happening.

Charles Adler is a professor of neurology at the Mayo Clinic-Scottsdale and one of the scientists featured in Owen's article. Adler's specialty is disorders that involve abnormal body movements such as those that occur with Parkinson's disease. It is interesting to note that in regard to his research on the yips, if you go to his laboratory's website, the third sentence of the background and rationale section reads:

"Golfers all know about the 'yips,' a term used to describe golfers who miss key putts in tournaments (recently mentioned as happening to Tiger Woods at the Masters)." Adler then goes on to cite studies that put the development of the yips in professional golfers as high as 30 percent. Another subject of *The New Yorker* article is Sherry Crews, a sports psychologist who acted as chair of the World Scientific Congress of Golf. She commented to Owen that "anxiety can exacerbate the yips—just as it exacerbates the tremors in Parkinson's disease—but it's not the cause, since the yips are usually present whether the yipper is nervous or not." Nevertheless, this begs the question, if someone on the tour does take Xanax or another anti-anxiety drug: would that be giving them a competitive advantage by minimizing the effect of the yips? Or if the yips truly is an underlying condition like Parkinson's disease in this example, then taking medication to battle a preexisting medical condition would seem like their right as a patient.

The scary downside, however, is that just adding Xanax to a professional athlete's medication regiment can have fatal consequences. Nearly 30 percent of fatal opioid overdoses in the general population involve benzodiazepines, of which Valium and Xanax are part of the family. Studies of methadone programs in Spain and Switzerland have found about half of those in the opioid dependence treatment program were also using benzodiazepines. In the Veterans Administration (VA) Health System, it has been found that nearly 30 percent of veterans were given overlapping prescriptions of opioids and benzodiazepines, which predictably resulted in an increased risk of death.

Eric Sun is a Stanford anesthesiologist and pain medicine expert with a PhD in Business Economics. Like most doctors, he was concerned by the increase in opioid-related deaths, especially those that were brought on by mixing or overlapping prescriptions for opioids and benzodiazepines. While most physicians know that prescribing the two medications together can be risky, Sun was under the impression that nonetheless, the prescribing of both medications had increased over time. That increase in overlapping prescriptions could potentially be contributing to the opioid epidemic. Therefore, he and his fellow researchers turned to the Marketscan Research Database. Marketscan is a deidentified (anonymous) database of patients enrolled in private insurance plans through a participating employer, health plan, or government organization. Over time, this database has grown from six million to over 35 million beneficiaries. Sun was able to identify 315,428 patients who filled at least one prescription for an opioid between 2001 and 2013. The group then cross-referenced the prescription list with emergency room visits or inpatient admissions for opioid overdose.

What they found was that the percentage of opioid users in the ER who had been coprescribed benzodiazepines nearly doubled from 9 percent in 2001 to 17 percent in 2013. That's an increase of almost 90 percent. Now, the reason the combination is so dangerous is that both drugs can suppress the signal for you to breathe, and when combined, they can actually overpower your brain's inherent signal to keep breathing. To Sun, these findings were important, because they showed a significant percentage of opioid overdoses could be stemming from doctors' overlapping prescriptions. According to his published work, "The practice of prescribing both medications had increased during the past decade, and moreover, in the population we looked at, we found that prescribing both medications was behind about 15% of hospitalizations for opioid overdose." In other words, 15 percent of people who were hospitalized for opioid overdose had overdosed in the setting of overlapping opioid and benzodiazepine doctor prescriptions.

The authors suggested that based on their data, elimination of concurrent benzodiazepine-opioid use could reduce the risk of emergency room visits related to opioid use by about 15 percent. It's fair to say, though, that most of these overlapping prescriptions aren't prescribed together on purpose. Without an accurate database of which prescriptions a patient has filled, it may be hard for a physician to know which medications someone is already using. In terms of Tiger's 2017 arrest, Dr. Sun had some thoughts: "I think his case just highlights the underlying risks to patients when they use both drugs simultaneously. Another common combination that is similarly risky is opioids plus alcohol." Sun goes on to provide a warning based on his years of studying pain and medication use: "Tiger is lucky that law enforcement—and not EMS—are the ones who found him."

In 2009, when Tiger crashed his car during a domestic dispute with his wife while under the influence of medications, celebrity gossip websites shed a light on Tiger's possible prescription drug problem. Then, in 2017, when Tiger was arrested for driving under the influence of prescription drugs, his mug shot and arrest video were plastered all over the news and the Internet. Public shaming was not, nor has it ever been, an effective method of inspiring change. Instead, Tiger sought professional help. Even legendary Olympic swimmer Michael Phelps, who had his own substance abuse struggles, reached out to help Tiger. He saw Tiger's DUI as a "massive scream for help." The pain medications were a simple fix that led to a major problem—the starlings effect of the professional athlete world. One year later, however, Tiger has undergone professional treatment for substance abuse dependence. And now, he has won the Masters Tournament for the first time in over a decade. Tiger finally addressed the problem in a deeper sense than a superficial Band-Aid. After years of spinal pain and a dependence on pain medication to play, and even despite his aging body, it's quite possible that Tiger's back.

References and Sources Used

LISTED BELOW ARE THE MULTIPLE references and sources I have used for each chapter of this book. Much of this information is in the public domain or accessible via subscription services. I would like to personally thank all of those individuals that provided personal communication via email or telephone. I would also like to thank the intrepid reporters and journalists out there whose work has helped educate me even further on these important events, whether from initial event reporting or looking back a decade or more later. These publications include newspaper articles, magazine articles, and online stories. Further, I would like to congratulate the authors whose published studies were used as references for this book, as their work is clearly well done. In any instance where a quote or reference is not made in the body of the book, the article may be found here.

Introduction

Siebert, Horst. *Der Kobra-Effekt. Wie man Irrwege der Wirtschaftspolitik vermeidet.* Munich: Deutsche Verlags-Anstalt, 2002.

Sandy Koufax, Tommy John, and an Epidemic

Grossfeld S. "Now campaigning against Tommy John surgery: Tommy John." *Boston Globe*. June 11, 2018.

Pendergast T. "Koufax: It Hurts Like Heck". *Santa Cruz Sentinel*, Vol 108, Number 97, April 23, 1964, Page 11.

Associated Press. "Cardinals Down Los Angeles 7-6; Koufax leaves game after first with torn muscle." *New York Times*, April 23, 1964, Page 46.

Verducci T. "The Left Arm Of God." *Sports Illustrated*, July 12, 1999.

Ahmad CS, Grantham WJ, Greiwe RM. "Public perceptions of Tommy John surgery." *Phys Sportsmed*. May 2012; 40(2): 64–72.

Conte SA, Hodgins JL, ElAttrache NS, Patterson-Flynn N, Ahmad CS. "Media perceptions of Tommy John surgery." *Phys Sportsmed*. Nov 2015; 43(4): 375–80.

Gibson BW, Webner D, Huffman GR, Sennett BJ. "Ulnar collateral ligament reconstruction in major league baseball pitchers." *Am J Sports Med*. Apr 2007; 35(4): 575–81.

Jiang JJ, Leland JM. "Analysis of pitching velocity in major league baseball players before and after ulnar collateral ligament reconstruction." *Am J Sports Med*. Apr 2014; 42(4): 880–5.

Makhni EC, Lee RW, Morrow ZS, Gualtieri AP, Gorroochurn P, Ahmad CS. "Performance, return to competition, and reinjury after Tommy John surgery in Major League Baseball pitchers: a review of 147 cases." *Am J Sports Med*. 2014; 42(6): 1323–1332.

Erickson BJ, Gupta AK, Harris JD, Bush-Joseph C, Bach BR, Abrams GD, San Juan AM, Cole BJ, Romeo AA. "Rate of return to pitching and performance after Tommy John surgery in Major League Baseball pitchers." *Am J Sports Med*. 2014; 42(3): 536–543.

Electronic personal communication with James Andrews as well as his book *Any Given Monday*. New York: Scribner, 2013.

Electronic and phone conversation with Jeff Passan

Electronic communication with John Manuel.

The Magic and Cookie Johnson Effect

Vann MG. "Of Rats, Rice, and Race: The Great Hanoi Rat Massacre, an Episode in French Colonial History." *French Colonial History.* 2003. Vol 4: 191–203.

Shilts R. "Speak for All, Magic." *Sports Illustrated.* November 18, 1991.

Friend T. "Still Stunning the World 10 years later." *ESPN The Magazine.* November 7, 2001.

Cote K. "AIDS and The No Fear Factor". Contribution by Ken Rodriguez. *Chicago Tribune.* March 31, 1996.

Palmer DA, Boardman B, Bauchner H. "Sixth and eighth graders and acquired immunodeficiency syndrome: the results of focus group analysis." *J Adolesc Health.* Oct 1996; 19(4): 297–302.

Tesoriero JM, Sorin MD, Burrows KA, LaChance-McCullough ML. "Harnessing the heightened public awareness of celebrity HIV disclosures: 'Magic' and 'Cookie' Johnson and HIV testing." AIDS Educ Prev. Jun 1995; 7(3): 232–50.

Centers for Disease Control and Prevention (CDC). "Sexual risk behaviors of STD clinic patients before and after Earvin 'Magic' Johnson's HIV-infection announcement—Maryland, 1991–1992." *MMWR Morb Mortal Wkly Rep.* Jan 29, 1993; 42(3): 45–8.

Ehde DM, Holm JE, Robbins GM. "The impact of Magic Johnson's HIV serostatus disclosure on unmarried college students' HIV knowledge, attitudes, risk perception, and sexual behavior." *Journal of American College Health.* 1995, Vol 44(2), pp.55–58.

Brown BR, Baranowski MD, Kulig JW, Stephenson JN, Perry B. "Searching for the Magic Johnson effect: AIDS, adolescents, and celebrity disclosure." *Adolescence* 1996, Vol. 31 (122), pp. 253–264.

Casey MK, Allen, M, Emmers-Sommer T, Sahlstein E, Degooyer D, Winters A, Wagner AE, Dun T. "When a Celebrity Contracts a Disease: The Example of Earvin 'Magic' Johnson's Announcement That He Was HIV Positive." *Journal of Health Communication,* Volume 8, pp. 249–265, 2003.

Marin G, Marin BV. "Perceived credibility of channels and sources of AIDS information among Hispanics." *AIDS Educ Prev.* Summer 1990; 2(2): 154–61.

Warren T. "Star Power." *Marketing Health Services.* Summer 2010, Vol 30, Issue 3, pp. 16–19.

Ayers JW, Althouse BM, Dredze M, Leas EC, Noar SM. "News and Internet Searches About Human Immunodeficiency Virus After Charlie Sheen's Disclosure." *JAMA Intern Med.* Apr 2016; 176(4): 552–54.

ESPN 30 for 30 documentary: "The Announcement"

Lyle Alzado and the Steroid Conversation

"Increased Outbreaks Associated with Nonpasteurized Milk, United States, 2007–2012." CDC Report.

Albright, MB. "Black Market Raw Milk—Healthy or Harmful?" NationalGeographic.com. May 5, 2014.

Neuwirth, R. "The Shadow Superpower." *Foreign Policy.* October 28, 2011.

Wendle, A. "Why Some States Want To Legalize Raw Milk Sales." NPR/Harvest Public Radio. February 20, 2015.

Schneider, F. "Shadow Economies and Corruption All Over the World: New Estimates for 145 Countries." *Economics*, July 9, 2007.

Medina L, Schneider F. "Shadow Economies Around the World: New Results for 143 Countries Over 1996–2014." 2017 Discussion Paper, Department of Economics, University of Linz, Linz, Austria.

Schneider F, Buehn A. "Shadow Economy: Estimation Methods, Problems, Results and Open questions." *Open Economics.* 2018; 1:1–29.

Assael, S. "Steroid Nation: Juiced Home Run Totals, Anti-aging Miracles, and a Hercules in Every High School: The Secret History of America's True Drug Addiction." ESPN (press). October 23, 2007.

"A Football Life—Lyle Alzado." NFL Productions. November 21, 2014.

Huzienga, R. *You're Okay, It's Just a Bruise.* New York: St. Martin's Press, 1994.

Alzado, L. "I'm Sick and I'm Scared." *Sports Illustrated.* July 8, 1991.

United Press International. "Former All-Pro Lyle Alzado dies, claimed steroids killed him." UPI Archives. May 14, 1992.

Zimmerman P and King P. *Dr. Z: The Lost Memoirs of an Irreverent Football Writer.* Triumph Books. September 1, 2017.

Kotler, S. "Sympathy for the Devil." *LA Weekly.* July 28, 2005.

Farrey, T. "The Memos: A Ban Ignored. *ESPN the Magazine.* Nov, 2005.

Hiserman, M, Munoz, T. "Playing a Dangerous Game : Drugs: Former Cal State Northridge player is a convicted cocaine dealer who used steroids. Now he is playing for Barcelona of the WLAF, hoping for another NFL opportunity." *LA Times.* March 18, 1992.

Personal Interviews: Chuck Yesalis, John Romano.

E-mail correspondence: Matt Chaney.

Len Bias and "Biased" Drug Laws

European Commission. "Proposal for a Regulation of the European Parliament and of the Council on the Common Fisheries Policy— general approach." 2012 11322/12.

Condie HM, Grant A, Catchpole TL. "Incentivising selective fishing under a policy to ban discards; lessons from European and global fisheries." *Marine Policy.* 2014; 45 (C): 287–292.

Condie HM, Catchpole TL, Grant A. "The short-term impacts of implementing catch quotas and a discard ban on English North Sea otter trawlers." *ICES Journal of Marine Science.* 2014; 71(5): 1266–1276.

Cronin, D. "Lack of quotas allowing EU fleet to decimate fish stocks off Africa." Politico. July 3, 2002.

Heath MR, Cook RM, Cameron AI, Morris DJ, Speirs DC. "Cascading ecological effects of eliminating fishery discards." *Nature Communications.* 2014; 5: 3893.

Guillen J, Holmes SJ, Carvalho N, Casey J, Dörner H, Gibin M, Mannini A, Vasilakopoulos P, Zanzi A. "A Review of the European Union Landing Obligation Focusing on Its Implications for Fisheries and the Environment." *Sustainability.* 2018; 10: 900.

Ungrady, D. "Send Len Bias to the Hall of Fame." *Washington Post.* June 17, 2011.

Salon. Interview with Eric Sterling June 19, 2011, Transcript at http://www.wbur.org/npr/137302172/op-ed-bias-death-prompted-shoddy-legislation.

Vagins, DJ (policy counsel for civil rights and civil liberties), McCurdy, J. (legislative counsel). "Cracks in the System: Twenty Years of the Unjust Federal Crack Cocaine Law." ACLU. Oct 2006.

Cloherty, KJ, Perlman, DM. "Powder vs. Crack." *Fed. Law.* March/ April 2003.

US Sentencing Commission, Special Report to Congress: Cocaine and Federal Sentencing Policy, 156, 161 (1995).

Chin, GJ. "Race, The War on Drugs, and the Collateral Consequences of Criminal Conviction." *Gender Race & Just.* 2002; 6: 253.

Becket, K. *Making Crime Pay: Law and Order in Contemporary American Politics.* New York: Oxford University Press, 1997.

2011 Report to the Congress: Mandatory Minimum Penalties in the Federal Criminal Justice, Chapter 8: Mandatory Minimum Penalties For Drug Offenses (2011).

Eric Sterling, personal interview.

Sumter Daily Item, Jan 15, 1983.

Time magazine, September 22, 1986.

Newsweek, June 16, 1986.

Hank Gathers, Dale Lloyd, and Athlete Screening

Berensondec, A. "End of Drug Trial Is a Big Loss for Pfizer." *New York Times.* December 4, 2006.

Hensley, S, Winslow, R. "Demise of a Blockbuster Drug Complicates Pfizer's Revamp. Failure Is a Blow for Promising Heart-Disease Treatment After Deaths in Trials." *Wall Street Journal.* Dec. 4, 2006.

Diep, F. "Cholesterol Conundrum. Changing HDL and LDL levels does not always alter heart disease or stroke risk." *Scientific American*. November 1, 2011.

Joy TR, Hegele RA. "The failure of torcetrapib: what have we learned?" *Br J Pharmacol*. Aug 2008; 154(7): 1379–1381.

Brousseau ME, Schaefer EJ, Wolfe ML, et al. "Effects of an Inhibitor of Cholesteryl Ester Transfer Protein on HDL Cholesterol." *N Engl J Med*. 2004; 350: 1505–1515.

ILLUMINATE Investigators. "Effects of Torcetrapib in Patients at High Risk for Coronary Events." *N Engl J Med*. 2007; 357: 2109–2122.

Madsen CM, Varbo A, Nordestgaard BG. "Extreme high high-density lipoprotein cholesterol is paradoxically associated with high mortality in men and women: two prospective cohort studies." *Eur Heart J*. Aug 21, 2017; 38(32): 2478–2486.

Drooz A., "Gathers Faints, but Kimble's 51 Keep Loyola From Collapse." *LA Times*. December 10, 1989.

Almond E, Drooz A, Hudson M, Robbins D. "LA Times: A Special Report." April 1, 1990.

ESPN 30 for 30 documentary: Guru of Go. 2010.

Medcalf M. "Hank Gathers, 25 years later." ESPN.com. Mar 4, 2015.

"Bo Kimble: Chris Bosh return 'not worth the risk.'" *SI* Wire. May 23, 2016.

Langford C. "Rice U, NCAA & Creatine Shake Blamed For Ballplayer's Death." Courthouse News Service. Courthousenews.com. September 24, 2008.

Zarda B. "NCAA to Screen for Sickle Cell." *USA Today*. July 1, 2010.

Bower M. "Parents of former Rice DB file wrongful death suit." *Houston Chronicle*. September 24, 2008.

Abkowitz JL. "President's Column—Sickle Cell Trait and Sports: Is the NCAA a Hematologist?" *The Hematologist*. May–June 2013, Vol 10, Issue 3.

Maron BJ, Friedman RA, Kligfield P, et al. "Assessment of the 12-lead ECG as a screening test for detection of cardiovascular disease in healthy general populations of young people (12–25 Years of Age): a scientific statement from the American Heart Association and the American College of Cardiolog." *Circulation.* 2014; 130: 1303–1334.

Email conversation with EKG-screening expert Kimberly Harmon.

Ayrton Senna, Dale Earnhardt, and NASCAR's Car of Tomorrow

Russeth A. "Harold Rosenberg Created Smokey the Bear." *Observer.* April 19, 2013.

Grennan R. "Getting the Hat Right: The Untold Origin of Smokey Bear." The University of Illinois Archives. August 23, 2013.

Donovan G, Brown T. "Be Careful What you Wish For: The Legacy of Smokey Bear." *Front Ecol Environ.* 2007; 5(2): 73–79.

Parkes I. "Ayrton Senna: The one positive from Senna's death has seen safety improvements prevent any further deaths in F1 20 years on." The Independent British online newspaper. April 30, 2014.

Taylor S, "Lunch with . . . Professor Sid Watkins." *Motor Sport Magazine.* September 13, 2012.

McGee R. "Thanks for the memories, CoT." ESPN.com. Feb 15, 2013.

Brudenell M. "NASCAR top executive in Detroit: We'll 'make mistakes."

Detroit Free Press. March 19, 2015.

"Schrader Discusses Earnhardt Crash." *LA Times.* Associated Press. March 15, 2001.

Waltrip, M. *In the Blink of an Eye: Dale, Daytona, and the Day Everything Changed.* New York: Hyperion Books. 2011.

Hinton E. "Earnhardt's death a watershed moment." ESPN.com. Feb 7, 2011.

Pulver DV. "Earnhardt's death changed racing." *Dayton Beach News-Journal.* Feb 18, 2011.

Paulsen. "Daytona 500 Finishes With New Record-Lows. Least-watched Daytona 500 on record." SportsMediaWatch.com. Available at: https://www.sportsmediawatch.com/2019/02/daytona-500-ratings -record-low/.

"Hello halo: Thong-like safety device divides F1." *Hurriyet Daily News*. March 20, 2018.

Personal Interview: Jon Mills.

Duk-koo Kim and Boxing's Biggest Tragedy

Robinson DL. "Do enforced bicycle helmet laws improve public health? No clear evidence from countries that have enforced the wearing of helmets." *BMJ*. Apr 2006; 332 (7545): 722–725.

Cycling to work in Melbourne 1976 to 2011. VicRoads Bicycle Project Team.

Jacobsen PL. "Safety in numbers: more walkers and bicyclists, safer walking and bicycling." *Inj Prev*. 2003; 9:205–9.

Carpenter CS, Stehr M. "Intended and Unintended Consequences of Youth Bicycle Helmet Laws." *The Journal of Law & Economics*. Vol. 54, No. 2 (May 2011), pp. 305–324.

Walker I, Robinson DL. "Bicycle helmet wearing is associated with closer overtaking by drivers: A response to Olivier and Walter, 2013." *Accid Anal Prev*. Feb 2019; 123: 107–113.

Kriegel M. "A Step Back. Families Continue to Heal 30 Years After Title Fight Between Ray Mancini and Duk-koo Kim." *New York Times*. September 16, 2012.

Kriegel, M. *The Good Son: The Life of Ray "Boom Boom" Mancini*. New York: Simon & Schuster, 2013.

Carp, S. "It Was a Brutal Fight." *Las Vegas Review-Journal*. November 13, 2007.

Wiley R. "Then All the Joy Turned To Sorrow." *Sports Illustrated*. November 22, 1982.

Agence France-Presse. "The tragic title fight that changed boxing." November 6, 2012.

Haberman C. NY Times Retro Report. November 8, 2015.

UPI. "Kim's Kidneys Are Removed." *New York Times*. November 19, 1982.

Boone D. "The Characters of Boxing." https://bleacherreport.com /articles/123538-the-characters-of-boxing-tex-cobb.

Vecsey G. "Sports of the Times: Cosell says 'I've Had It." *New York Times*. December 6, 1982.

National Association of Attorneys General Boxing Task Force. May, 2000.https://ag.ny.gov/sites/default/files/press-releases/archived/report .pdf

Jetton AM, Lawrence MM, Meucci M, Haines TL, Collier SR, Morris DM, Utter AC. "Dehydration and acute weight gain in mixed martial arts fighters before competition." *J Strength Cond Res*. May 2013; 27(5) :1322–6.

Gelber JD, Cohen A, Wallace P., "Do Weight Classes Matter? Weight Cutting and Performance of Professional Mixed Martial Arts Fighters and Boxers." Unpublished data.

Conversations with veteran ringside physicians Paul Wallace, Margaret Goodman, and Joe Estwanik.

Tom Brady and Protecting the Quarterback

Davis LW. "Saturday Driving Restrictions Fail to Improve Air Quality in Mexico City." *Scientific Reports*. 2017; 7: 41652.

Munoz SE, Giosan L, Therrell MD, Remo JWF, Shen Z, Sullivan RM, Wiman C, O'Donnell M, Donnelly JP. "Climatic control of Mississippi River flood hazard amplified by river engineering." *Nature*. Apr 4, 2018; 556 (7699): 95–98.

Layden T. "The Roughing the Passer Rule and Football's Unfixable Problem." *Sports Illustrated*. October 8, 2018.

Goff B. "The NFL's Quarterback Protection Problem." Forbes.com. September 27, 2018.

Gasper CL. "Brady rule: Steps taken to protect QBs' knees." The *Boston Globe*. March 24, 2009.

Binney Z. "Weight and Injuries." March 15, 2018. https://www .footballoutsiders.com/stat-analysis/2018/weight-and-injuries.

Reid J, McManus J. "The NFL's racial divide." ESPN's The Undefeated. https://theundefeated.com/features/the-nfls-racial-divide/.

Eisen, R. *Total Access: A Journey to the Center of the NFL Universe*. New York; St. Martin's Press, 2008.

Mullins L. "The Oral History of Joe Theismann's Broken Leg." *Washingtonian*. October 2015.

Clark MD, Varangis EML, Champagne AA, Giovanello KS, Shi F, Kerr ZY, Smith JK, Guskiewicz KM. "Effects of Career Duration, Concussion History, and Playing Position on White Matter Microstructure and Functional Neural Recruitment in Former College and Professional Football Athletes." *Radiology*. Mar 2018; 286(3): 967–977.

Lewis, M. *The Blind Side*. New York: W.W. Norton and Company, 2006.

TIDES 2018 NFL Racial and Gender Report Card: National Football League. Available at: https://www.tidesport.org/racial-gender-report-card.

TIDES 2015 NFL Racial and Gender Report Card: National Football League. Available at: https://www.tidesport.org/racial-gender-report-card

"NFL Season By Season Team Offense." ProfootballReference.com. Available at: https://www.pro-football-reference.com/years/NFL/index.htm.

Paulsen. "A Closer Look at the NFL's Long, Bad Season." SportsMediaWatch.com. February 9, 2018. Available at: https://www.sportsmediawatch.com/2018/02/nfl-ratings-decline-2017-analysis/.

Tiger's Back

Kelly J. "In the 1920s, Washington had birds on the brain." *Washington Post*. September 29, 2015.

Zielinski S. "The Invasive Species We Can Blame On Shakespeare." Smithsonian.com. October 4, 2011.

O'Brien J. "The birds of Shakespeare cause US trouble". BBC.com. April 24, 2014.

Carlic S. "Introducing America's most hated bird: The Starling." The Associated Press. September 7, 2009.

Reints R. "Throwback Thursday: The Worst Bird Strike in U.S. History." *Boston Magazine*. October 5, 2017.

"Tiger Woods Arrest Report." *New York Times.* May 30, 2017.

Holmes J, "Tiger Woods drops to ground with back spasms at The Barclays". PGA.com. August 25, 2013.

DiMeglio S. "Tiger Woods withdraws from Honda Classic with back spasms." *USA Today.* March 2, 2014.

Callahan M. "The night Tiger Woods was exposed as a serial cheater." *New York Post.* November 24, 2013.

Murray E. "Tiger Woods admits that latest back problems have curtailed his powers." *The Guardian.* March 9, 2014.

Cottler LB, Ben Abdallah A, Cummings SM, Barr J, Banks R, Forchheimer R. "Injury, pain, and prescription opioid use among former National Football League (NFL) players." *Drug Alcohol Depend.* Jul 1 2011; 116(1–3): 188–94.

Dunne EM, Striley CW, Mannes ZL, Asken BM, Ennis (formerly Whitehead) N, Cottler LB. "Reasons for Prescripion Opioid Use While Playing in the National Football League as Risk Factors for Current Use and Misuse Among Former Players." *Clin J Sport Med.* Jun 28 2018.

Pennington B. "Heart Medications May Also Calm Nerves, Keeping Them Banned." *New York Times.* November 14, 2012.

"Substance list, testing has some PGA golfers fuming." Associated Press. January 29, 2008.

Perkel C. "Anthony Galea, sports doctor to elite athletes, loses licence for nine months." The Canadian Press. December 6, 2017.

Benedict, J, Keteyian, A. *Tiger Woods.* New York: Simon and Schuster, 2018.

"Almost a quarter of PGA Tour pros surveyed by *Sports Illustrated* think Woods took PEDs," Golf.com. May 13, 2010.

The 2017–2018 PGA Anti-Doping Manual. Available at https://www .usga.org/content/dam/usga/pdf/2018/2017-2018_Anti_Doping _Manual.PDF.

Schlabach M. "Tiger and the Masters victory even he never saw coming." ESPN.com. April 14, 2019.

Owen D. "The Yips. What's behind the condition that every golfer dreads?" *The New Yorker.* May 19, 2014.

Charles H. Addler laboratory: https://www.mayo.edu/research/labs/parkinsons-disease-movement-disorders/yips-focal-task-specific-dystonia.

Madden P. "The PGA Tour's Drug-Testing Policy Needs a Big Fix." Golf.com. January 27, 2016.

Crouse K, Pennington B. "Panic Attack Leads to Hospital on Way to Golfer's First Victory." *New York Times.* November 12, 2012.

Sobel J. "Beljan learning to deal with panic attacks." Golfchannel.com. January 3, 2013.

Sun EC, Dixit A, Humphreys K, Darnall BD, Baker LC, Mackey S. "Association between concurrent use of prescription opioids and benzodiazepines and overdose: retrospective analysis." *BMJ.* Mar 14, 2017; 356: j760.

Fernández Sobrino AM, Fernández Rodríguez V, López Castro J. "Benzodiazepine use in a sample of patients on a treatment program with opiate derivatives (PTDO)." *Adicciones* 2009; 21: 143–6.

Meiler A, Mino A, Chatton A, Broers B. "Benzodiazepine use in a methadone maintenance programme: patient characteristics and the physician's dilemma." *Schweiz Arch Neurol Psychiatr.* 2005; 156: 310–7.

Park TW, Saitz R, Ganoczy D, Ilgen MA, Bohnert AS. "Benzodiazepine prescribing patterns and deaths from drug overdose *among US veterans receiving opioid analgesics: case-cohort study.*" BMJ2015;350:h2698.

Jones JD, Mogali S, Comer SD. "Polydrug abuse: a review of opioid and benzodiazepine combination use." *Drug Alcohol Depend.* 2012; 12.